All The Footprints In My Sand

By

Tracy Hunt Casey

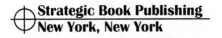

Strategic Book Publishing
New York, New York

Strategic Book Publishing
An imprint of AEG Publishing Group
845 Third Avenue, 6th Floor—6016
New York, NY 10022
www.StrategicBookPublishing.com

ISBN: 978-1-60693-154-7
SKU: 1-60693-154-7

Printed in the United States of America

Book Design: Roger Hayes

Dedication

For Mom

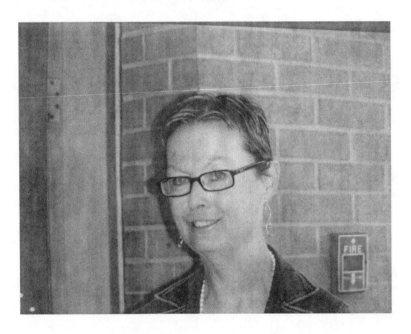

Forward

On November 19, 2005, for her 54th birthday, I gave my Mom a journal and a pen. She had forever wanted to write about her fight with cancer. On the inside of her card, I wrote, with my husbands help, "The written word is every person's opportunity to live forever. Here's your opportunity mom, write away."

I got that journal back from my father upon my mother's death. I was excited to open it, but when I did, all the pages were still blank. My heart sank. For whatever reason, Mom couldn't write her feelings down; maybe the fear of facing it and seeing it in writing scared her. She wanted to call her book "Spirit."

I started this journal to help me cope with her loss. It seemed right that I use the journal I gave her to write through my feelings and keep in touch with her through my writing. I unknowingly began a journey I had no idea I was about to take, as a result of a gift she had given me. I didn't know two years ago how this simple pure hearted journal would one day be my book, my "spirit."

I started writing the day she died. Now, two years later, as my personal journey has ended, I have compiled all my thoughts and feelings along the journey that I shared with my mom, knowing that, though my mom could never write about her life, I needed to write about mine; two years of sorrow, of pain and recovery, but always with the will to move forward.

Thank you, Mom.

All The Footprints In My Sand

On May 11, 2006, my mom passed away. Her three-year battle with cancer had finally ended. She was my mentor, my loudest cheerleader, my conscience; Diane Margaret Hunt, now gone in her 54th year.

In the fall of 2005, before she died, she took a test that gave me, her eldest daughter, the greatest gift of all, the gift of foreknowledge that would save me and all future generations in my family from ever having to fight the same battle she did, so bravely, so proudly, for so long.

Monday, August 21, 2006, was the day that saved my life. The day I was informed that I had inherited the BRCA1 genetic mutation from my mother. Having this mutation predisposed me to breast cancer at an 85% likelihood, and ovarian at 44%. But all I heard was that my life had been saved, in my mother's death.

As I read stories, books, and obituaries of women lost to breast cancer, a common word is always used: courage. I don't believe this is the word I will use with my mom, although it was used in her obituary, "...she fought a courageous battle..." Isn't courage when you have the choice to fight? She had no choice; she had to fight. There was no other option, but she had an attitude — a positive attitude — and I believe it was this positive attitude, this "it could be worse" attitude, that allows our loved ones who fight this fight to last longer, change some outcomes, and leave strength in the ones left behind. This is the courage I guess many speak of; the courage not to give up, and to continue to live. In reality, they do have a choice; to let it stop them, to stall their life, or to do what they can to live as long as they can.

My mother's greatest legacy to me was her positive attitude. I never realized how strong her attitude to overcome the worst scenarios was, until I witnessed her in her gravest battle.

This book was written to inspire, and to allow others going through a similar situation to share in my journey, and through it, gain something they didn't have before — something to help get through it and make the decisions that are best for you. I want to help others see the other side of it. Maybe you know someone who has gone through what I have; it gives you eyes into their journey, so you may better understand it and better support and love them through it.

The BRCA1 gene is known to be responsible for a small percentage of breast cancer. This may be due, in part, to the lack of knowledge about it: when to get tested, how to go about it, who to ask, and then, what to do about it.

This book is not to tell you to go out right away and do the test, or get a prophylactic mastectomy and oopherectomy, as I did. It is my therapy, my closure and my way of honoring my mother's gift, her strength, to let the world know that Diane Hunt lived here, and my journey these past couple of years and to honor and thank all the footprints in my sand. I say this and titled my book as I did because of the famous poem "Footprints." A copy was given to me by my Mom. It was found on magnets, bookmarks, and key chains. It is a poem of one feeling alone at the darkest hour, walking along the beach and then, when looking back only seeing one set of footprints, assuming it was their own. When they pray to God and ask where God was in their hour of need, God says, I carried you during that time; it is my footprints you see.

One thing this journey has shown me is that there were many footprints in my sand, not just one. Many were there to carry me through, in different ways, and this book, is also to recognize and thank them all.

ৡৱ ৡৱ ৡৱ

I started a diary on May 11, 2006, the day my mom died. Why? At the time, I needed to vent. I needed to talk to her, to work through it, as I was overwhelmed with sadness. I remembered hearing it was good to write feelings down, and to still be close to her. Now, writing keeps me close to her. Even two years later, I talk with mom. She still brings me objectivity and closure and direction. As I reflect back on my thoughts a couple days later, I have clarity that I didn't have before. I still have mom listening, just on paper, but I will take it. And I remember her clearly as ever; this journal has given me that. As time went by and I realized I had the BRCA1, I needed her. No one else would or could possibly understand what I was about to go through, not even me.

ৡৱ ৡৱ ৡৱ

Throughout this book, I will reflect back and insert some of my journal conversations with Mom.

I hope this book will enlighten, inspire, and encourage you to do things you may have been afraid to do, to demand knowledge and act on it, and most importantly, to know that whatever may be going on in your life, it could be worse. Feel it, go through it, and then move off of it toward resolution; the quicker the better. Life is too short.

HER DEATH

Journal Excerpt: May 11, 2006 7:30 a.m.

The phone rings earlier this morning, my husband, who owned his own business was out delivering drawings. My kids are still in bed, ready to get up for school any moment.

I answer, it's my sister Tammy.

"Tracy, remain calm, mom stopped breathing and EMS is at the house".

I start pacing and shaking and crying "oh my God oh my God oh my God," is all I can manage to get out.

"TRACY, calm down, and meet me at dad's house"

I tried calling my husband on his cell phone, he had taken my car, I had his there, I don't know why I just didn't take it, I wasn't thinking straight, I could have loaded up the kids taken them to the daycare and then gone to dad's, but no, I had to wait, keep calling and wait.

かゝ かゝ かゝ

His cell phone was a busy, I called his office, busy called his cell, busy, his office, busy still. Oh my God oh my God mom is dying and I need you where the hell are you?

かゝ かゝ かゝ

I called his coworker at home, not home. Called his cell again, he finally answered, its mom, its mom I need you here now, where are you, get here now. I'm coming down the road, I'll be there. Oh my God, oh my God oh my God, okay, focus. Kids. They need breakfast, get dressed, get them dressed give them breakfast. I finish all of this and run out up and down the driveway waiting, helpless. I call his cell again, where the hell are you? He finally pulls in the driveway, he gets out I get in after what seemed hours later.

Mom, I am coming, hold on for me, I am coming.

I called my boss, I won't be in to work, called my best friend for support, called my dad.

Dad, I am on my way, what's happening, he says they took mom in the ambulance meet us at the hospital, I am waiting for your sister to come pick me up. Okay,- dad, is mom going to be ok. No said dad, sobbing. I am sobbing.

Still thinking mom was alive but not for long, I raced panicked to get to the hospital before she died. I don't even know how I got there when I did. I parked and ran to emergency where dad said she would be. I lived 20 min from the hospital. Dad lived 5 min.

"Tracy", said an officer, who I recognized from high school, called out to me. He escorted me to a small room, asked where my dad was. I thought he'd be there all ready since I lived further away.

I said he's coming. He said "first I want to express my sincere condolences. Your mother has passed away." At first I thought, he is mistaken, how did he know who my mother was? He confirmed her name. I was wrecked. I need to see her, maybe I should wait for Dad and Tammy, no :I need to see her, I said. "Okay follow me" he said.

As I followed the officer, I didn't know what to expect, I was so overwhelmed with shock and sadness. As I entered into where they had her in emergency, there she laid covered to her neck in blankets, mouth open, eyes closed, hair off her face. I laid over her, held her hand kissed her ran my fingers through her hair that fell out with every caress, so I stopped.

"I'm here mom, dad is coming, I'm here, I love you mom, I miss you so much I 'm so sorry I wasn't here sooner

11

I'm so sorry I couldn't tell you one more time I love you. you were so brave mom you went the way you wanted you were so tired. I love you mom you were a good mom, oh mom. I held her hand rubbed her belly rubbed her hand kissed her I could hear her say "where is your father?" and then I could hear him and my sister coming in.

"Dad, Tammy" we all embraced sobbing uncontrollably. She's in no more pain, she's better where she is she went the way she wanted. She loved you dad, she loved you girls. As they stood over mom, I called my husband to come.

"Rick, moms dead", "she's dead?", I am so sorry Tracy I am so sorry Tracy. I am on my way.

Dad went to use the phone to call a family friend to help make calls. He contacted the funeral home and our family minister. We were all in the room again sobbing when Rick arrived. We were all just sobbing. A social worker kept coming in to offer support and counseling none of us needed or wanted her there, we need to be alone. Mom had been sick fighting this breast and ovarian cancer for 3 years, the last couple of months she was steadily deteriorating. The chemo that had sustained her last year had stopped being effective as the cancer had adapted to it. Since January, she had been on 3 different chemotherapies, none of them working.

I saw my mom last on the Tuesday only 2 days before her death with Tammy.

Mom had to have shots regularly for low iron and this Tuesday arranged for the first time in three years to have them done at home. She couldn't make it to the hospital anymore. Mom was weak, tired, and immobile from chemo, the cancer and her drastic weight loss left her resembling an Ethiopian person starved from hunger, skin and bones, literally.

But she still had her laugh, her voice, her wisdom, her love, she was still Mom.

That Tuesday, Tammy and I decided to surprise her as we usually took her to get her shots, (we did all her treatments together), but she said we didn't need to be there. We wanted to comfort her as we knew it was a very hard thing for her to admit she couldn't do it anymore, to admit she was getting worse.

We arrived at 930am a half hour before the nurse was to come. We went to the front door as she had it opened all the time so she could still see what was going on in the outside world (she was actually nosy and wanted to keep up on what the neighbors were up to!)

"Hi what are you doing here?" she said in her high pitch happy tone. "we came to keep you company for your first home shot!' we said. "Oh that's so nice, thank you."

Mom was 54 years old, but she looked 90. She was thin and frail except for her protruding belly from the acetes, a symptom of ovarian cancer.

That day seemed no worse to me than any other day. I didn't notice anything worse. The only indication of something that caught my attention of concern was her very very low blood pressure, I saw it concerned the nurse, as she stated it was very low, and I could see my mom was concerned as well. The nurse said she would notify the cancer clinic and asked my mom if she had the number, mom said she didn't know it, which I knew was a lie as she called it daily almost. I knew she was afraid they would admit her, after the nurse left I stayed for a bit and then Tammy and I left her.

"Before you go can you pick up those bits under the table, get my sticky roller and use it to get them, this table your dad made me keeps dropping bark as it dries out!"

"Aw, yes mom" (she always had us pick up bits whenever we came over, so it was annoying at this point, sick or not, she is still mom!) The bit was my mother's nemesis since I can remember. She was forever vacuuming them, sweeping them and mopping them up…what is a bit anyway? Well if you were to ask my mom, it is the tiniest particle seen only by her eyes, but to which you need to pick up, even though you can't see this bit, she can, and since she couldn't get them up anymore regularly, we were now the bit catchers!!! I kissed her on my way out and hugged her bony frame, but I felt the warm peach fuzz on her cheek as I hugged her, a feeling that I long to feel again to this day. I dream of it regularly.

As I was leaving something told me to stay a little longer, another hour even, my next appointment for work wasn't until the afternoon, but I wanted to get to Walmart to buy the kids some clothes for the warmer weather, they had outgrown all the ones from last year.

Now, as I stood in the room where she was lying, I wished with all my heart I would have stayed, I wish I would have listened to that voice, I vowed, from that moment on, I would.

I tried to make myself feel less guilty, even if it was 5 years from now, I'd still want one more hour, one more day. I called her daily to check in and told her I loved her everyday, I would share funny stories from work with her everyday, but in this moment, it wasn't nearly enough. I should have stayed.

⁊₰ ⁊₰ ⁊₰

We stayed with her in that emergency room until blood started to pool around her chest area. We stayed in that room until her hands went porcelain white. We stayed in that room until we had to leave to go to the funeral home that afternoon. We couldn't leave her. We didn't want to leave her. We stayed for a few hours after she had passed.

But it wasn't long enough for me. I needed to feel her touch, I felt comforted just seeing her body there even though I'd known she had been long gone, hopefully with her dad, whom she loved very much.

ৰ্জ ৰ্জ ৰ্জ

My mom was 54 years old, woke up one Thursday morning at 7am not being able to breath, my dad awoke and called 911 against my mom's wishes. He didn't know what to do. He called 911 she needed oxygen. He performed CPR, he laid her down told her to get some rest, help was on the way and that he loved her very much. He said they shared a look between them that they both knew this was the moment and in that moment my mom was done with her fight, she died at home with her husband, just like she wanted.

ৰ্জ ৰ্জ ৰ্জ

I am 35 years old, planning my mother's funeral, is what had ran through my head as I sobbed in the washroom at the funeral home sitting on the toilet.

It was all so surreal.

THE FUNERAL

At the funeral home we were planning for the funeral, it was like I was outside myself looking in on it almost. So many times I went through this in my head over the past three years. Mom had told me and Tammy what her wishes were two years prior in the Golden Griddle during breakfast, our Monday morning after chemo ritual. I always looked forward to Monday mornings, (note to those out there going through chemo: attach something positive to the day, as we did, it was our family breaky day.). I still remember where we were sitting what I was eating and how I reacted — by crying, as I always did when we talked about it, I am a very sensitive and highly emotional person.

☙☞ ☙☞ ☙☞

Those requests came back clear to me today. She wanted to wear her Hawaiian dress that she got in Hawaii five years earlier. It was the best trip of her life and favorite time with my dad. She wanted songs like Danny Boy, Amazing Grace, Psalm 23 and Billy Joel's, "River of Dreams." This song meant something to her from her first battle ten years prior.

She wanted her friend and pastor to do the ceremony with his wife, and she wanted to be cremated. She wanted the cancer burned out of her.

She told me she hadn't told dad any of this, as she didn't think he would remember when the time came, and didn't want him to have that pressure of remembering. That day, when I dropped her off at home, I repeated it all in my head so I would never forget. I never wrote it down, I didn't have to.

We wrote her obituary, something I had already written many times in my head and on paper but today I wasn't supposed to be, and would do anything not to be. Seeing her death in words a few short hours after it happened seemed too fast. Her visitation would be the next day with her funeral following the day after, and her burial not till the following week as her pastor wasn't available until then, and she wanted him to perform the interment.

I left the funeral home sadder than I have ever been. I got a tingling feeling in my jaw that didn't go away until after her burial. Dad said it was nerves.

HUNT: Diane Margaret:

After a courageous battle with cancer, Diane Margaret Hunt (nee Rodney)

Passed away peacefully on Thursday, May 11, 2006 at age 54 years. Much loved

Wife of Thomas "Tom" Hunt for 36 years. Much loved mother of Tracy Casey and her husband Richard of Scotland, and Tammy Eechaute and her husband Mike of Brantford. Loving grandmother of Emily and Jack Casey, Austin and Alyssa Smith and Riley Eechaute. Loved by mother-in-law Irene Hunt. Dear sister-in-law of John Hunt and his wife Carolyn, Doug Hunt and his wife Katie and Valerie Hunt. Dear aunt of Jonathan and Megan Hunt. Diane will be missed by many loving friends at Brant County Ford and Five Oaks, and previously at Echo Place United Church and the Brantford Expositor. The family expresses sincere thanks to Dr. Chouinard, the oncology nurses and staff at the BGH, and Rev. Paul Fayter, friend and pastor his wife Lily, for their support and care over the last 3 years.

Friends and relatives will be received by the family at MCLEISTER FUNERAL HOME, 495 Park Rd. N. on Friday from 6pm until 9pm and Saturday from 2pm until 3pm, and are invited to wear something pink in her memory. The funeral service will be in the chapel Saturday at 3pm, followed by cremation.

Rev. Paul Fayter will officiate. In lieu of flowers, memorial donations to Five Oaks United Church Education Centre or the Cancer Society gratefully appreciated.

కా-ళ్ళి కా-ళ్ళి కా-ళ్ళి

Dad, Tammy and I are now the Three Muskateers, he says. At this point we go home we all sleep in their house getting pictures together for the next couple of days. We all go to bed crying and all woke up crying, the same time mom woke up the day before, not being able to breathe and dying.

We can't believe she has gone so quickly. We all know it is what she wanted (to die at home peacefully) but we weren't prepared, although we all believed we were before. We now know we are not prepared for life without mom, wife, Diane. We pull together to get each one through it. We don't fight; we hug like mom would have wanted. I take care of the paperwork part, and Tammy takes care of the thanking people. And Dad, dad is dad, unfocussed, fidgety and dazed, truly sad and lost.

All that has gone through my head since mom died is her telling me to take care of Dad, as she believed I would be handling most of it, to watch out for Dad, make sure he didn't become a workaholic, and that he didn't get taken advantage of by women with ill intentions! All of this from the moment I knew she was dead is still going through my head a week later. But I will get there.

❧❧ ❧❧ ❧❧

My next entry in my journal isn't until June 1. As I look back as I am writing this book, I regret I didn't write about the funeral. However, I know I was deeply upset and could not bear to write it down. It was hard for me to write about the day of her death, as it is hard even now.

I still remember, now two years later, how she looked, the people who came out, and the fear of going on without her. I also remember reading from *These Days*, a publication for the Presbyterian Church. Mom had submitted some writings that reflected scripture in the Bible when she worked for the United Church. They liked what she had submitted, and she was given a week's worth in the book to write some inspiring scripture for the publication, and relate it to something in her life.

I found this booklet upon searching through her things days before for the funeral. I always knew about it and she had given us all a copy, however, when I opened it, Mom's writings were for the week of May 12-18! She wrote this back in 1996. Was it prophetic of what we needed to hear the week of her actual death ten years later? If Mom could find a way to reach us, she would. This was her way. I had to read it.

I read her scripture and her inspiring story for May 13, the date of her funeral ten years later, and I wondered if what she wrote would have relevance for me to read at her funeral. Did it ever! This was Mom's writing, her words. She probably had no idea we would need to hear them so much on this day, or that they would be read on the day of her funeral.

Wonders and Warnings (from "These Days,"
1996, Diane Hunt)
"When it is evening you say, "it will be fine
weather, for the sky is red." And in the morning, "it

19

will be stormy today, for the sky is red and threatening." You know how to interpret the appearance of the sky, but you cannot interpret the signs of the times."
Matthew 16:2-3

The black clouds were forming in the grey skies above us. The dense smell of the air told us of impending doom. Suddenly, the winds began to stir. Birds were taking flight. All indications said, "Head for shelter!" We had just settled in for a relaxing day of leisure and didn't want to turn back. We waited, too long.

"Attention!" bellowed the official on the Coast Guard cutter. "Engage your engine, and I'll guide you to shore. There is a tornado warning in effect."

Nature has its way of surprising us every day. What seems to be obvious at the time of setting out on our daily journeys of life can be changed in an instant. Nothing's for sure. But if we kept the faith, it will sustain us in times of turmoil and trouble as well as in good times.

This was what we needed to hear: that although we did not expect this, we had to keep faith that we could go on without her, knowing she was with us always. It reminded us to live in the moment, as things could change so quickly, as mom did for the last three years. She relished every moment with us, and left nothing unsaid.

She spoke at her own funeral.

Journal Excerpt: June 11, 2006

It has been one month since your passing and it still feels like you died this morning. I tried to keep busy today with my family, Tammy visited your grave and Dad went to Toronto with friends to a motorcycle show.

We are redecorating Dad's bedroom, he is getting rid of your waterbed — you loved that bed, but it is too hard for Dad, you took your last breaths there.

He is feeling a lot of guilt about your death that morning, wondering if he should have done more to try to save you. Regretting not being in the ambulance with you and waiting for Tammy. I know I wish he was there too. I still remember I could hear you in that emergency room wondering where the hell Dad was, as was I , you always asked, "what is he doing?" in your tone that Tammy and I will remember always!

Tammy and I went to Walmart yesterday and both of us remembered you telling us to park at the front and leave you the keys while you waited as we ran in to get what you had requested. Everywhere I go, I can recall us there, a call I had with you, or an errand I ran for you. Dad wants your clothes cleaned out. I want to do it as I would like some of your things, I fit into your clothes. But I can't bring myself to do it Mom. I remember you today on the Sunday before you died, you weren't doing well. We sat on my couch, you held me and my hand, you just wanted to sit with me quietly, did you know you were dying? You tried to eat what you could, and then left, and driving away in the truck you blew me a kiss and mouthed the words "I love you" to me through the window as you were driving away, you were wearing your cream arctic fleece coat and the hood was on your head , you were cold a lot. I took a snapshot of that moment that is engraved in my memory, I remember saying to myself remember that, it could be the last time I see you, I do that a lot lately, trying to remember every kiss, every hug. I still cry a lot. I was your eldest daughter, I love you so much and must have known your struggles and that is why I was good growing up Mom. I didn't want to bring you more hardship. I only wanted to bring you joy. I always wanted your approval, always wanted you to be proud of me. Anything I did in life I always wondered what decision would make you and Dad proud, my high school classes, my grades, my friends, my boyfriends, my university, my first car, my first house, my husband…

The only decision I made without your blessing or input was me moving home 3 ½ years ago when Dad called me with the bad news of your diagnosis. I never hesitated selling my house and moving my family. Although I liked it there Mom, I knew you loved coming up, but I loved you more and wanted no regrets. I know you were happier after I was home for a while.

Mom I need to know you are with me, I really need to know. I ask you every night and day do something to let me know you are happy where you are that you are watching over me. I need that, I am ready for that.

I miss you, I still need you.

Love

Tracy xoxox

Journal Excerpt: June 23, 2006

Mom, today I had a dream about you. I was in a crowded room in a house and I looked over and saw you sitting in the corner in an easy chair in the same exact outfit you were wearing at your funeral. You had your wig and your glasses on too. I came over to you balling, not believing you were there and I tried talking to you but it was noisy so I grabbed your hand and led you outside. I was sobbing, sobbing, hugging you sooo tight telling you how much I missed you, and were glad that you came back. I told you all about Dad and asked you if you were proud of me and the way I have handled things.

You laughed your laugh and said you were always proud of me and that you couldn't worry about Dad anymore and that Tammy and I had to stop doing things for him. You called to grandpa at one point. I asked you if you were happy where you were and I can't remember exactly, but I think you said you weren't in heaven yet, you were still on your way there. You also said if I ever needed to see you that I could just go to where we were now, that exact place —outside that house on the back porch (or did you mean in my dreams?) and you would always be there for me.

☙❧ ☙❧ ☙❧

Mom, I don't know if that was really you, but it is the second dream I have had of you saying similar things. I hope it was you because I still need to see and feel you and I really felt your hug. If you are hearing me or able to ready my thoughts, I want you to know I felt that hug so much it resonates on my body as I write this. I am going to record every time I dream of you coming to me.

Mom, I still miss you so much. I still can't believe it. Just as I think the worst of the grieving is over, I am whipped back into it like a bungee cord. I have a scarf and a

23

hat of yours that still have your scent on them, I am going to smell them right now. I love you. Thank you for taking care of all of us.

I love you.xoxoxox
"Tracy tree"

ABOUT DIANE

Born on November 19, 1952, an only child to Dorothy and Vogan Rodney, unwanted by a jealous mother, and the apple of her alcoholic father's eye, she was raised in an emotionally absent and physically abusive home. Mentally by her mother, and physically by her father. When he would come home drunk, her mother would yell at him, tell him all the bad stuff my mom did that day, and tell him to take care of it.

My mother forgave her dad. She said she believed it wasn't really his fault, that it was his disease that made him do it. She loved her dad; she tolerated her mom.

This is when the first appearance of my mom's attitude came to me. She could have become her mother or her father; however, didn't. She took another path. Her dream was only and always to have a family of her own — her definition of family, not the one she lived.

She wanted her family to have lots of love for each other, respect and openness and honesty. She didn't aspire to be a great doctor, or teacher; she wanted to be a great mother. And she was.

She stayed home and raised my sister and me. My father pumped gas before I was born and then became a mechanic. We were raised and supported on his income alone. It wasn't until I was in grade 6 that mom took a part-time job, sorting flyers at the local newspaper.

We could always count on dinner together every night (roast beef dinner on Sundays), her constant need to vacuum the "bit" daily, and her being involved in our school activities, be it our education or troubles with friends. Her family was always her priority and we knew it.

She lost her dad when I was in grade 3. She lost her mom when I was in university. After her dad died, her mother made my mom purchase anything she wanted of her Dad's. Her mother wouldn't give it to her. She then gave the car my dad wanted to her hairdresser, and my mom had to beg for items she wanted. They had no money; my dad was only breadwinner, and her mom knew that. She was punishing her now that her dad wasn't around to protect her.

This was the other time my mother rose above a hardship and moved forward in her life. She also began to write after her father's death, as I did after she died. It helped her to remember him.

I found a poem that Mom had written in calligraphy, framed, and tucked away in a drawer. This was the poem she wrote about her dad. This, too, was read at her burial, as again, it was so prophetic. It was Mom's words, and we needed to hear from her now.

> *Beneath the surface guarded and protected*
> *Lay golden memories etched into our minds*
> *Like pages in a photo album*
> *Reminders of the good times and the sad...*
> *Not yet a one ever goes unnoticed*
> *All the little mentions that were you*
> *Sacrifices that were gladly given*
> *Without a thought to what might lie ahead*
> *When always rising to the call of duty*
> *No regrets about the choices ever said*

Instead you marched the distance to the finish
Remaining loving, loyal, strong and true
That's why of all my treasures I hold dearest
Cherished deeply is the one I have of you.

It was like Mom had written exactly how I had felt about her. I wept when I read it, and we all sobbed at her burial when I read it again. Mom was speaking to us, loving us, and there for us, helping us to get through, from beyond.

ᐁᐧᐃ ᐁᐧᐃ ᐁᐧᐃ

I can't imagine her losing the one parent whom she loved and loved her back, and then having to contend with this. I was thankful to have a caring, loving father to support me through the loss of my mom.

My mom held few jobs in her life. Her last and most accomplished was that of a car salesperson at a local Ford dealership. She just woke up one morning and something told her to go ask them for a job. She had never sold anything before in her life, and now she was going to ask them to hire her to sell cars. And they did!

She became a consistent top performer, who loved her team. And, her team loved her. It was her last place of work before she died. She tried to keep working as long as she could.

Her first bout of cancer was when I was in university; my first year. It was only a lump, and they did a lumpectomy and radiation, and she was good for ten years.

I wasn't there for my mom then. I was busy in university, starting a new chapter in my life and couldn't deal. I rarely went home, until one day I did, and found her home, bald. The cancer now had a face. It wasn't hidden deep under her skin where I couldn't see it, and could deny it easily. It was looking me right in the face.

27

And I crumbled. I went with her to a couple of radiation treatments, but that was it.

I think, when she was diagnosed again in 2003, I vowed I wouldn't leave her or Dad alone this time in the battle. I was older, had children of my own, and didn't want any regrets.

THE CANCER CALL

It was April in 2003. I was living about two hours north of Mom and Dad. I had just had my second child, my son, five months earlier, and my daughter was three.

I remember getting a call from my mom. It was at night. She told me they thought she had lung cancer. How was that possible? I didn't understand. She didn't smoke ever, my dad didn't smoke ever, and she didn't work in a workplace where there was smoking.

My dad was too weepy to talk. She told me she had found a lump in her breast weeks earlier but did nothing about it as she thought it was scar tissue from previous radiations and biopsies so she ignored it. She then developed what she thought was pneumonia. When she went to the doctor and had an x ray done, there was fluid building in the pleural lining of her lungs. This caused them to believe originally that it was lung cancer.

A couple of days later she had a mammogram. There it was: breast cancer. The cancer had spread to her body fluid and was building in her lungs as it couldn't escape.

She was stage 4 in April of 2003.

In anger and sadness for this disease, anger at my mom for not getting it checked sooner, wondering how she could have left it so long, to sadness that I am going to lose my mom to cancer. We sold our home, and moved home to be closer to her for what time we had left, as we all thought it was imminent. I thank you, Rick, to this day, for supporting me in that major decision.

I was on maternity leave, so it was easy to do the move. I would just ask for transfer. Mom was the important thing right now. Rick got a new job, and we found a house to rent so we didn't have to rush and buy something in haste.

She couldn't believe I up and sold my house! She was angry at first because she loved coming up. She called it her cottage! But I had to do it. I knew she wouldn't be able to come up as much and I knew I needed to be there more than I was ten years prior.

In the two years that followed, my mother had 22 peracenteses procedures (when they remove the liquid buildup in her pleural lining), and a mastectomy with only a local anesthetic. She opted for this way, as she refused through her whole illness to stay overnight in the hospital. She did each procedure as a day surgery to avoid staying overnight. She was afraid she would never leave. She remembered her father being admitted and never leaving. He died at the hospital, alone with only the nurses around, and she didn't want that. She had a plan. She wanted to stay at home — and what Mom wanted, Mom got. She had a very strong, sometimes stubborn, will.

She had many thoracenteses performed as well, where they drained the fluid from her abdomen. She got to be so big, we used to ask when she was expecting! She made a joke of it, made light of her side effects and her disease. That helped us all get through it.

She never talked of her death, never asked the doctor for her prognosis, and never wanted to hear the "worst case" scenario. All she wanted was quality of life for the time she had remaining. It was an attitude her doctor picked up on, and he never gave her anymore info that what he knew she needed to go on fighting and living.

There were many times I wanted to and was invited to go and talk to her doctor about her illness and her prognosis, but I felt I would be betraying the wish of my mom. So we all did it her way, knowing the day would come, however, not knowing when.

She used to say that we could all die any day, we were all going to, we could get hit by a bus getting off the curb, no one ever knew their time, as she didn't. She just knew it was cancer that would take her. However, in the end, she believed it would be her heart that would just give out, just get tired and stop. And it did.

It was her last bout of chemo that I saw fear and realization that the time was nearing. He prescribed a strong dose of chemo, which was very hard on the heart, and because she had been fighting three years, her heart was already weak. She had already lost over 100 pounds. She feared this last chemo, as she believed it would harm her heart, but she trusted her doctor and he had taken her this far. It was from February, 2006, that she went down quickly.

My mother was a very heavy woman when she was diagnosed. She fought with her weight all her life. It was a symptom of her upbringing, I believe.

But I also believe that if she wasn't heavy, we would have lost her much sooner. It was this weight that allowed her to fight longer. It almost cushioned her through the chemotherapies. She could afford to lose it, and as she became closer to 100 pounds, it took its toll quickly.

I asked her only once if she was afraid, as I couldn't muster up the emotional strength for her reply. It would hurt me to hear my mom say that she was scared. We were in Dairy Queen parking lot for our weekly ritual of hot dog with mustard and chocolate shake, extra chocolate.

I asked her if she was scared. This was in her first year; my son was a baby, sleeping in the back seat. She said of course she was afraid, but she believed in God and heaven and had accepted it, that she couldn't focus on dying, and had to focus on living, and inspire hope in us. She said she was very graceful on this journey to her light, and didn't want to leave us, of course, but God needed her. She had done what she was meant to do here.

❧ ❧ ❧

During her illness, I had to take a leave from my career. I was suffering from what my doctor told me was anticipatory grieving, grieving her death before her death. I was always thinking about her dying, her funeral, when it would be. I had always prayed to God to take her at home in her sleep, let her heart stop and her be with dad, not alone at home in the afternoon. I never knew then that my prayer would be answered on the morning of May 11, 2006.

Due to the stress I was under, I was advised to take time with her by my doctor while she was still alive to enjoy, so I did. I spent the summer of 2005 with my mom.

❧ ❧ ❧

I have to sidebar here. I work for the greatest company in the world. A company that is for women, and that practices what it preaches. I was a district manager with Avon Canada at the time, had been with them for five years. I had the greatest support from a team of women, my sister managers in Niagara, Gail and Marcia to name a couple, who were key to keeping me striving for more at work, and my Division Manager, Linda, who carried me and supported me during this time, no questions asked. For that, I am eternally grateful. Avon gave me a valuable, irreplaceable gift. In the years that followed with my personal journey, they were always supportive and caring. They mentored me and always supported my dream of moving forward in the company and my personal dreams. I wish everyone could work for a company like mine (oh, but wait, you can!).

This company everyday allows me to help and coach women from any walk of life, to change their lives, and to feel better, whether it means putting on a lipstick or building a career. I am not trying to preach here, but I really do believe we are a great company, and I am so blessed to be a part of it. But now, instead of coaching, I had to live what I had been coaching all along. To keep going get over this hurdle and to move on.

This company was meant to be my career. They are a huge financial supporter of research and education for breast cancer.

I was living it, and they were working on raising funds to eradicate it. It was a great partnership. When I was hired in 2001, I had no idea the importance it would have in my life. You see, they had a profound effect on my life, and still do. They are some of the footprints in my sand.

ॐ॰ॐ ॐ॰ॐ ॐ॰ॐ

During this summer off, mom would come and pick me up, even though I lived twenty minutes away. We would go do errands, banking, always went to Shoppers Drug Mart. She loved that store (for sticky rollers! She couldn't vacuum much but the sticky roller could pick up those bits just as easy!), and the grocery store. I would run in with her list, but not before she went over it with me, like when I was young. And when I came out with everything, she would go through list again to ensure I had everything! I remember her always doing this when I was young; some things never change! Whatever Tammy or I did for her, we did it the best! It was her way to encourage us (oh, you are the best at that! Thank you!). The best part of doing errands with my mom was you always got to keep the change!

Then we would have lunch at her one of her favorite places. She didn't eat much. She had this trick that she thought fooled us; she would move her food around on her plate and sometimes put an empty fork in her mouth and say, "mmmm!" She didn't have much of an appetite with the chemo. We always had a Timmies in hand, and laughs were endless.

She had the best laugh. Everyone who knew her knows this. It was infectious, and you knew it was her when you heard it. These days it was followed by a cough or two afterwards, which my sister can imitate well now! We never talked about cancer that summer; we just enjoyed each other. She knew why I was off. She was supportive and worried about me, and she didn't want to be the cause of any depression. I reassured her it wasn't her, that it was about Rick's business troubles with his partner. I think she bought it, or maybe she just let me think that. I went back to work that September.

৵৽ ৵৽ ৵৽

It was a rollercoaster ride, those three years. She would have great remissions, where she would look her best, and go back to work. We would all get our hopes up and then the chemo would not work anymore and she would have to change, and she would be on a downslide again. Many times in these downslides, we all thought this was it, and then she would rebound. It was emotionally and mentally draining. Cancer affects everyone close to you, differently than the person going through it. I can't speak the viewpoint of someone fighting it, only the viewpoint of the daughter on the sidelines.

I went through many stages; anger, a lot of anger, regret, sadness, a lot of sadness to the point of melancholy, and bartering with God. But I always got through by obtaining information and I vowed to have no regrets when the time did come. I left nothing unsaid. She truly knew how I felt about her, her love for me and mine for her, and her positive impact on me and my life. The information I sought would be about every chemo she was on, every pill and shot, and what the next steps were to be. I would go online and investigate. I have always been a believer of knowledge being power. I always loved school, right through to university. I love learning; it helped me to cope, and to grow with life.

I needed knowledge, and Mom knew this. She did not; she had faith. But she let me do my research and would want to hear only about the treatments she was on, no prognoses. It wasn't until the fall of 2005 that she started to get ascetes in her abdomen, some bleeding and abdominal pain and feeling of being full all the time

ॐॐ ॐॐ ॐॐ

Immediately I thought ovarian cancer. She did not. At her appointment the following day, I asked her doctor to do a CA125 test. My mom didn't know I was going to do this and didn't even know what the test was. I found information online that it measures the levels of the cancer antigen 125, which is a protein that is found at levels in most ovarian cancer cells that are elevated compared to normal levels. This test would give us an idea if we were dealing with ovarian cancer, as I believed we were. I believe it said anything over 35 U/ml is abnormal. Mom's test came back in the hundreds.

We were now dealing with a second cancer, one I believe was there long before her breast cancer, and had gone undetected through the past couple years due to her treatments. The two were separate cases, the doctor said. My mother couldn't believe it, and couldn't believe the doctor didn't pick up on it or do a test with her symptoms. She was now upset and scared, and wondered how the hell, she now had two separate cancers to fight, how she was going to do it. Her doctor started her on chemo for the ovarian, as the breast cancer and fluid in her lungs was at bay. Now was the time to attack to ovarian cancer.

I knew that ovarian cancer was hereditary, so I started to do some research into genetic testing. I found out about the genetic inheritance of certain diseases and that breast cancer was genetic in some cases. In doing further research, I discovered the BRCA1 and the BRCA2 mutations.

In the fall of 2005, I asked my mom if she would take a DNA test. She had always wondered why she got the cancers, what she did or did not do to get it. It was an unanswered question to which this test might give her the answer. She was reluctant at first, as she didn't know what it entailed. I knew there was a family history of ovarian cancer in her family, but we weren't aware of any breast cancer.

I told her it was a simple blood test, but first she needed to do paperwork. She hated paperwork! She asked her doctor for me. Even though I know she didn't really want to do it; she was doing it for me. Her doctor set up the genetic counseling appointment. She filled in a family tree health history as best she could. She had to go back three generations and was shocked after doing it the best she could at how prevalent cancer was in her maternal line. After she submitted that, they determined there was a chance of it being hereditary. A couple months later, she got a call and she took the simple blood test in that same fall of 2005, six months before she passed away.

In February of 2006, we got the answer. My mother was BRCA1 positive, without a doubt, 100%. They said it was rare to get a true positive on a test like this. It meant there was no doubt she had the BRCA1 mutation. This meant she had inherited these diseases. She got her answer. She didn't inflict this on herself. My only regret is she didn't have the resources or foreknowledge she gave me. She died three months later, but in her death, unbeknownst to her, she had given her eldest daughter life, for a second time.

ॐॐ ॐॐ ॐॐ

You may be asking what prompted me to start this search. Through my life, I had followed my mother's health history to a "t." It was like I was a "mini" Diane Hunt. I knew if she got this test done and it was positive, that I would be. I just knew. I truly was my mother's daughter!

So on that day in February, in the chemo clinic that we found out it was positive, I had to excuse myself, and began crying down the hall, knowing I was next, not knowing the prevention yet.

My dad followed me, tried to calm me down, saying I wouldn't get it, I would inherit the "crazy" gene, if any, from his side of the family, trying to get me to laugh.

I washed my face and had to stop crying. My mom was in the other room getting chemo for Christ sake, it wasn't about me. But in that moment, it was.

As I went back to meet Mom, she was angry. She said, "You were the one who wanted me to take the damn test, why are you upset? I only did it for you. I never would have done it." I apologized. I didn't want her to be upset or worry about me. She needed to fight more.

In the weeks that followed, Mom said that Tammy and I would be seeing a genetic counselor at McMaster and go through the same process she did. However, it would take months.

Mom died before Tammy and I even got a call. We got the call two months after she died. She never knew, and my dad said he was grateful she didn't know, as it would have brought her pain and guilt for passing this on to one of us.

I never did or have blamed my mom. I have never looked at my diagnosis as her fault. I have always looked at it as a gift she left for me and my children and their children's children.

On August 21, 2006, we got our results. They were not shocking to me.

Journal Excerpt: August 21, 2006

Well Mom, today Tammy and I went for our results for our BRCA1 genetic test, I am 100% true positive which means I carry or have the same mutation you had which predisposes me to getting breast cancer at 85% likelihood; and ovarian 44% likelihood of getting it in my lifetime. They found the mutation on the exact same DNA strand that they found yours. Yours was like a road map and they just followed mine to the same spot, and there it was. Amazing what they can do now. I now am starting to see the results of the funds raised for breast cancer research.

We all went together mom, you'd be proud. To be honest, I expected these results. Tammy is negative, which is good it ends with her. Alyssa won't get it as it doesn't skip a generation. Now I am to go see an oncologist who specializes in this and then will see surgeons for double mastectomy and hysterectomy. I didn't cry mom, I was strong. I am looking at in as good news. I mean, mom YOU SAVED MY LIFE!!! You gave me an incredible gift of years with my children. If I didn't have this test, I wouldn't know and in 7 years I would be where you were 3 years ago. I thank you for doing that for me. I know you weren't too sure or all for it but you will be the last one this terrible disease takes of your children grandchildren and their children.

You were the bravest, strongest most guarded person I know and I will be the same way as I face these following months of consultations, and hard decisions of what path I want to take to ensure I don't get the cancer that took you from me. I miss you so much. I need a hug from you to tell me it will be ok, although I know and pray I make the right decision. Maybe its best you aren't here to know you passed it to your first baby, mom I in no way blame you at all. I thank you for doing the test for me I only wish you had done this test 10 years ago so you would still be here with me. I haven't let Tammy and Dad know how upset and scared I am. I don't want them to get upset. Dad is still in a fragile place and I don't want to load this on him. I know you understand that cause that's what you did with me and Tammy. I joked with Tammy saying if I did have a double mastectomy and didn't get implants that I could cut the grass with my shirt off!!! Ha ha!. Or I could get my dream boobs finally and dad could buy me my nipples!! For Christmas!!! And I don't want the cheapy style, I want the Harley Davidson of nipples! Tammy said I should get pancake nipples where the areola is most of my breast! I laughed so hard and I can hear you laughing too mom. Tammy and I can both hear it so clearly and it's comforting now.

I leave for Ottawa tomorrow for 5 days for Avon conference. Rick is coming on Friday to join me for the weekend. We need it, although I hate being away from the kids any long amount of time, I worry and hope that all is well when I am gone. Dad is taking Spanky and Jeanette is watching the kids and the cat. We painted our living room and hall you would love it! It is like from a magazine, actually it is. I copied it from a picture of a living room I liked and I did pretty good too! Everyone is impressed as am I! It's my best work yet! I did it to keep my mind off of today.

Anyway mom, I know I have lots of love and support from Rick, Dad and Tammy but I still miss the support that came from you. It was like no other.

I hope you come to me in my dreams throughout this difficult for me, just after you died, now I am faced with this!

Mom, again, thank you, seriously, and I love you but I mostly just miss you so much it aches and makes me feel sick inside. Deep inside my soul.

Love Tracy XO

WHAT IS BRCA1?

The BRCA1 is a genetic mutation located on a particular chromosome, 17q21, and is the gene responsible for increased susceptibility to familial breast and ovarian cancer *(Nature Genetics*, 22, 37-43, 1999).

A detailed family history to assess cancer risk involves collecting information with regard to types of cancer and the ages at which the cancer diagnoses were made. Also, the vital status of three generations of relatives in a family is needed.

The average woman has an 11% lifetime risk of developing breast cancer, and a 1.5% lifetime risk of developing ovarian cancer.

Women such as myself and my mom, with the BRCA1, have an 85% lifetime risk of developing breast cancer and a 44% lifetime risk of developing ovarian cancer. That was too high for me. I am not a gambler or a risk taker.

About one in 200 women in North America carries a BRCA1 or BRCA2 mutation.

Patients identified as being at increased risk for any familial cancers should be referred for genetic counseling. The Ontario Medical Review published guidelines for the referral of patients with a family history of cancer to cancer genetic clinics.

Information on genetic counseling centres within Canada can be found at http://www.cagc-accg.ca (Metcalfe,

Open Medicine, Vol. No. 3, 2007). In the United States to find a genetics specialist near you, call the National Institute for Cancer at 1-800-4-CANCER.

The value of this testing comes from reducing the number of women who develop breast cancer and the number of women who die from the disease. We now have more knowledge to conquer it where we can, earlier or totally. This is good news for that one in 200! Some signs that you may be at risk of carrying the BRCA1 are, breast cancer at age 45 or younger, breast cancer in both breasts at any time, breast and ovarian cancer in same woman, male breast cancer in the family, two or more in a family diagnosed with breast and /or ovarian cancer.

Women with the BRCA1 or BRCA2 mutation may consider several options for prevention. The three main options are prophylactic mastectomy (with optional reconstruction), prophylactic oopherectomy (removing ovaries, uterus, fallopian tubes, cervix), or chemoprevention (tamoxifen, raloxifene). In addition a woman may elect to undergo routine screening (secondary prevention) with the goal of detecting any cancers at an early, treatable stage. (Metcalfe, *Open Medicine*, Vol. 1, No. 3, 2007).

ॐ॰ॐ ॐ॰ॐ ॐ॰ॐ

On August 21, I found out about all of these options. I had some time to consider all my options and was set to visit Women's College Hospital to get more information. And on October 25, I had my first consult with my oncologist surgeon at the Jurvinski Clinic in Hamilton.

WHY DID I CHOOSE WHAT I DID?

This disease is very personal to many. How anyone overcomes anything in life is very different. Our coping skill level, our reasons, our life, all vary, so this book is not to encourage you to do what I did, but to make you aware of the options, and the journey I took with the personal decision I made based on my life.

At the time, I had two children, aged six and three. I was 35 years old, and had a great, successful career. I also had just witnessed how the cancer took my mom slowly over three years. I couldn't bear to go through what she did. I did not want my kids to have to witness that, if there was a sure way I could prevent it. The chemo drug was a no for me. There is no longitudinal study to determine the negative effects of taking these drugs indefinitely, and to do an MRI every year was too stressful for me. Every shadow would be investigated and biopsied, and most women, I was told, after two years are so stressed about it, they end up doing the prophylactic route anyway.

ক্ষ্ণ   ক্ষ্ণ   ক্ষ্ণ

The only sure way for me to get peace of mind was to opt for the mastectomy with reconstruction and the oopherectomy. I had my two beautiful children. My husband had a vasectomy and my periods were hell; this was not a major decision for me.

I opted for the mastectomy first, as my mother's first cancer diagnosis came when she was 42. My genetic counselor told me they had found that those with the BRCA1 who did get cancer presented ten years earlier, at times, in the next generation. I was already three years over my ten year mark. So I went for that first, with the plan of the oopherectomy to follow.

My mastectomy was set for March 2007. It was now October 2006. I had no second thoughts, no concerns. I was going to take this gift and run with it. What's that saying? Don't kick a gift horse in the mouth? I wasn't kicking!

In the months that followed, many things happened. One big thing was that my family bought a new home; a dream I had since selling ours in 2003 to move home to be with mom. The time was never right to buy. There was too much going on and my husband had decided to go out on his own in business. After a hard hit with his business (which is another book!), he went back to the company he was with before we moved. I had earned bonuses from my job and we had what we needed to finally buy our home! And we did in February 2007, one month before my mastectomy. We were to move in April 30, six weeks after my surgery! Many called me crazy. I call me ambitious! This was what I needed to focus on, to help me through this major surgery. I was about to lose my breasts; these babies fed my babies, brought me sexual satisfaction, and were a part of me, but let's face it, they were only boobs. They weren't a major organ. They didn't make me who I was, and heck, I could stand to get better, more perky ones out of the deal!

৵৶ ৵৶ ৵৶

So, we had the house happening, and we were packing. At this time, as well, with Avon, we were launching our tulip planting, (we are not just lipstick you know). We planted over 140,000 pink tulips across Canada, all paid for by Avon, and given to any organization that would support us in our quest to end this disease. In October 2006, we planted everywhere! Our job as managers was to find locations to plant these bulbs.

It was with this opportunity that I was able to give back to the hospital that gave my mom so much support, and a good quality of life for three years, the Brantford General Hospital. It was five months after Mom's death, and what better way to honor her and all the other women and families affected by this disease. I met with the hospital administration, and it was a resounding yes!

Journal Excerpt: October 18, 2006

Well, tomorrow we plant pink tulips outside the D wing at the hospital and we are planting them in the shape of a ribbon right along the walkway into the hospital. We have over 800 bulbs and will have hospital staff, patients and reps, friends and family planting for someone they love or lost to breast cancer. Avon is providing all these tulips across Canada. I am very proud. Mom I think you would have liked it and been proud of me. I have done this because of you and really for you I have just been given the vehicle through Avon to do it. I don't know how I will be, Dad and Tammy will be there. Maybe tough if your nurses come out to plant, but really want it to be a good day, not a sad day. I will let you know how it went. I go see the mastectomy surgeon on Oct 25. Rick can't go as he just started his job so I will be going alone. Maybe I will have Tammy go to, I don't know yet. It may stress me out more I think. I am sooo tired. Been running on empty. Hope I don't get sick, bad colds going around. Night, love ya. Come and give me some hugs soon.

XO Tracy

Journal Excerpt: October 20, 2006

We planted the pink tulips and we had a lot of support! Tammy and I were in the paper as was Five Oaks was mentioned as well. It was emotional for me when all the nurses from D wing came out. That's when I cried. Missing you. They said they miss you very very much too. Here is the weird part. On the day you died, I was outside of emergency crying getting some air, and a female security guard came up and offered tissue to me and to comfort me. Yesterday, we had a one more bulb to plant and there was a security guard by the main doors, a hospital staff called her over and mom it was the same woman! She was there the day you died and was the last one to plant a bulb! I felt better, leaving there yesterday than I ever have. I really felt like I did something. I know when I used to walk that way, before your chemo or drain, I hoped for strength for you mom, and when we left and walked out I prayed and hope that this chemo did it, that it would get it this time. And I wanted something along that same path, for women who were going in that they weren't alone going in — there were women with them and there were many hoping with them too. And it would inspire them to live and fight and hope and be courageous and brave like you were mom.

Today I also had my stitches removed. It was benign so no cancer in the lesion on my cheek. It is created by the nerve cells. I've had it since I had Emily. But mom, when I was in that room next door to where you used to have your abdomen drains, I wondered how you did it. I was just getting stitches removed, that pinched and felt ill after, but you had litres drained from you mom I don't know how you did it, with us all in the room with you, never flinching. But I think I do know why you did it and how you got through it, just the same as I will experience this next year. I will get through it because of my kids and that is the why and the how any women going through it, gets through it and continues the fight.

I don't know why but I want everyone to know about you and your strength through this I want to give others courage and positive outlook like you had. Plus I really want you to live forever, and if I do this you just aren't in my thoughts, it will be like you are alive again, mom. That's really what I want. For you to be alive again. Maybe if you went with your gut about being nervous about the last chemo you were on being hard on your heart he would have switched it and you'd still be here.

In your death you gave me a model of strength and courage that a women can get through it and I will get through it I just really need you here when I go into that hospital I want my mom there. I am starting to get a little scared because next week is my first appt with the mastectomy surgeon. Nothing will happen till next year I know. I want to be in my own home to come home to. I want to earn the big year-end commission from Avon, Rick's business to be cleared up and my kids to have big bedrooms. I want to come home after all of this to my dreams. A stable career for Rick, a home and be healthy.

ই৵ৰ   ই৵ৰ   ই৵ৰ

The pain is still as strong and more, it hasn't lessened. Its like, as events occur that you should be here for, I miss you more. And everything I do, like rake the leaves or think of Halloween, or anything, I think, you were here for all of this last year, and now you aren't. They say the first year is the hardest for that reason. I think dad is having his moments too. I think once the snow comes and there's not much to distract him he will have a tough time. His birthday is coming up and Christmas and he's buying gifts this year and doesn't have a clue! Tammy will do it like she did for you when you were sick!

Love you Mom, you inspire me every day.

XO Tracy

Journal Excerpt: November 13, 2006

I dreamt of you last nite. I think because yesterday was Emily's 7th birthday and we watched the video of the day she was born. I was so happy too when I saw your face and heard your voice mom. I have longed to hear your voice since you died and since dad asked me to erase your voice off the answering machine. I think those are the two things I miss most, your hug and your voice. No matter how sick you got, always hugged and always spoke the same way you always did. I can still remember it.

I dreamt last nite about my upcoming operations. I am so torn on when to do them as my Avon will be doing so well I hate to sacrifice anything. I want to make circle next year finally and am in position to do so. I have to go in February and then I don't know. Maybe in May? July? The year seems so short when I have to plan time away! Plus I will have 3 weeks vacation to use up on top of my 4 weeks of recovery for each surgery, and I get my new vehicle early next year and I don't want to be away when I get that! I must sound so silly to you mom, I know I shouldn't wait a year, I couldn't, but I don't want to work like a dog anymore to make bonuses 2007 is truly my year for the trips, commissions, incentives, house, it truly is but I don't know how I will fit it all in.

You were by my bedside in the video, when I was in labor with Emily, I wished you could be by my bedside this time too. No one else would get it but you. Dad, Tammy mean well but I need you mom. I have gained 12 pounds since you died. I want to get in shape before and lose 20 lbs but I just can't get going! I have wanted to start walking each morning but just can't get motivated. I have had a crappy 3 years please I pray 2007 is my year for career and personal success. This year has been the absolute hardest. But I will survive and go on , one thing you showed me from your life is you can recoup from hardships and grow stronger and control the outcome to an extent.

Dads birthday is tomorrow mom, does he cry to you as often as I do? Does he miss you and talk to you as much as I do? I hope if you can see me that you are proud of me. I don't know why but I have always longed for your acceptance and recognition. I have always wanted to make you proud of me.

Don't forget to come and give me hugs and when I need to see and hear you and feel you next to me I will watch that video.

෭෧ ෭෧ ෭෧

In 6 days you would have been 55. We lost you too young you were so young, so sad. I am nervous about Christmas, I don't want to break down, where are you? Are you in heaven now?

It seems this journal should be more full than this in 6 months but unfortunately I talk to you more than I write! I am regretful of that but looking back through this journal I write to you weekly. I miss my house in Alcona, forgot to tell you. I can't wait to be a homeowner again.

Love Tracy XO

Journal Excerpt: December 21, 2006

Hey Mom. I saw you last night in my dreams. I was walking through a hotel lobby to the entrance and when the sliding doors opened I looked to my right and you were standing there in the corner. I remember you looked great Mom. Better than in all my other visits with you. You had a dark denim fitted suit on and you were thin and had makeup on and your hair was short and sassy!

I said, "Mom is that really you?" you walked over to me I had to touch your face I remember I touched it like I was blind! I remember putting my cheek to yours and feeling the soft thing peach fuzz on your cheek against mine. We didn't really say too much you told me no one else could see you so I would look crazy to onlookers talking and reaching to no one! I do remember a lady walking through and stopped and noticed I was wearing a silver ribbon necklace — the breast cancer ribbon and she commented on how beautiful it was and where I got it and how tragic a disease it was and how hard when we lose a loved one to it. I agreed and cried when she said that and then she left and I turned to talk to you and you were gone. I really need to believe it was really you mom, and I believe you are in heaven now. Because you looked so good and when I woke up this morning and remembered, for the first time I didn't cry. I felt as if you really are still here for me mom. However as I write this I am teary eyed.

Anyways, Christmas is 4 days away, I am doing Christmas Eve, Tammy is doing Christmas then we are going to Kingston for New Year. I love you mom.

Tracy XO

Journal Excerpt: December 25, 2006

Merry Christmas Mom. We had Christmas over here. Dad gave me and Tammy an ornament for the tree with your name on it and date of birth and death. I cried. Mom, he did really great this Christmas! He did for me and Tam what you would have done for us. I love him so much.

Went to Tammy's today all was great there too Doug did his magic show, Katie busy face painting kids, they loved that!

After everyone left I broke down in Dads arms. He was very consoling. We shared some tears Christmas Eve with the ornaments but tonite it was just me. I don't know how he could be so strong at Christmas. I think he was doing it for me it had to be hard for him waking up alone on Christmas. I had him come for breakfast. Mom I missed you. I kept thinking about what I would've gotten you how you would have been feeling your laugh your cough. Sometimes when I remember you it is surface like but other times I feel it deep down in my gut and can envision you right in front of me it is so strong and powerful that I feel sick inside cause I know it's not real. I tried to remember last Christmas how you were doing what I gave you what you gave me, and I had a hard time remembering. I know you were full on your belly but I think you were doing better it was March you really started to go down. I look back in that memory box you gave me for Christmas in 2004. It was when you weren't doing well, it is one of the best gifts you could have given to me Mom. I gave Dad a picture in a frame of me, Tam and him from when were where in Gr. 9 and Gr.6 at Niagara Falls! He doesn't have one of the three of us and I thought it would be nice for him. I wanted to make Tammy a scrapbook of all the Christmas pictures of you, but when I went to your house to find some all I did was cry and I couldn't do it mom. I have all the pictures of your reactions to the gifts you got throughout the years, I miss that, and how you would get your own gifts and wrap them and act surprised!!! How you always got Dad a watch!

I pray you are in heaven that you are well and happy and that you can still somehow connect with me. Dad is still doing the same things that you did together, I hate the thought of him being alone.

I love you Mom, missed you so much at Christmas

Tracy XO

Journal Excerpt: January 31, 2007

Well today is Tam's birthday. We celebrated on the weekend.

BIG NEWS!! Rick and I put an offer in on a house!!!!! I feel sick, excited and nervous! The bank pre-approved us and I have the down payment so now just waiting for acceptance of the offer! I am still nervous it might not happen.

You would like it! Chocolate ceramic floor in kitchen, quaker style cupboards, dark hardwood, nice carpet in basement, totally finished. 3 bedrooms plus one downstairs, 2 bathrooms, fenced yard and daycare in the new school just around corner!!! Its all brick with double garage and shed in back. its been on market for 5 mths I am shocked it hasn't sold! It's meant to be! I will let you know for sure bank gives final approval. I just hope they don't say no. Our banker said no worries, it's a go! Mom I know if you could make this happen you would! I hope you can! If anyone can influence someone it would be you! Give a whisper!

To be cont'd....I love you wish you were here to see it!

Tracy xo

Journal Excerpt: February 1, 2007

WE GOT THE HOUSE!!! The bank said it was the fastest approval they have ever had!!! (thanks) wink wink!

I believe 2007 is my year. I believed in the fall it was going to be. I will have my surgeries and then be in my new home end of April!! Kids are excited too! Love the house and the new school, its brand new too! Rick likes his job, I am going to Vegas with Diane next weekend!! Sooo excited for that!

Wish you were here to see it mom.

Love Tracy XO

WHAT HAPPENS IN VEGAS ......

My sister in law, Diane, who is also a very good friend of mine, called. She knew the stress I was under, and she was under some of her own. She called me one night, and said, "let's go to Vegas, let's get the hell out of here! Next weekend!" I can't believe it but I said yes. We booked it the next night online (I have never ever been that spontaneous) and our husbands were very supportive of it. We are blessed to have them. We were gone the next week, for three days only!! That trip was an awesome, restful pause from our troubles, a full-of-laughs trip, something we both needed, and while I was there a very strange thing happened to me.

We were in the New York New York casino, held over due to a bad snow storm Our flight that was supposed to have left that morning at 7am wasn't leaving until that night, so we took a cab back to the Vegas strip from the airport and hung out, our first stop the New York New York casino. They had a great Mexican restaurant with great nachos and margaritas! Diane went to use the bathroom in the casino and I waited for her by some slot machines. I looked over and a woman with a dark brown ponytail caught my eye, and motioned to come over to me. I thought she needed to use my cell phone as I was about to call Rick. She introduced herself and said, "This may sound odd but I was drawn here to you." She said she was a psychic from Nevada and was off today. She was in shorts and had a fanny pack!

She said while she was there she was being pulled by a force; someone from the other realm was telling her to find me. She had been walking around the casino looking for me, and she said when she saw my eyes she knew it was me. She asked me if my name was Tracy and if I would mind if she talked to me, no charge but she had a message for me. I was reluctant; thinking "what is this woman trying to sell me!"

At that moment, Diane came over, I told her what was going on and she said, "It's your Mom, Tracy, talk to her".

So I agreed and we sat in the casino at two slot machines side by side while she told me that my move was a good move. She knew about the house, she knew the type of work I did, and said there would be success for me in 2009 Then she started talking about my upcoming surgeries. I started crying, Diane was crying. She was specific, and told me I needed to do it, Mom was with me all the way, she loved me and was proud of me. I was making the right decision, she was always with me.

I have never had this type of experience ever or since. I was crying in the middle of New York New York casino in Las Vegas on a hot afternoon, and my Mom was there.

For those of you reading this that are skeptics, I hear you and understand, however, it truly did happen and before my mom died I told her to find anyway she could to let me know she was still around me. This was her way. She knew I was open to this kind of thing as I had gone to see a psychic years ago. This was the perfect time for her to contact me; I was open, relaxed and away from familiar atmosphere where there would be no doubt it was truly her. Some of you who have had experiences like mine know you are not alone in this. They feed our souls at that time. Real or imagined, they are what help us to get through. We take what we need from them to help us overcome the tragedies in our lives.

That experience has stayed with me. Diane and I were in awe. We couldn't stop talking about it and I am glad she witnessed it.

That was a couple weeks before my mastectomy, and she knew I needed her. I am so glad I went on that trip, Diane, thank you!!

Journal Excerpt: February 27, 2007

Hi Mom. Pretty emotional couple of days. Grasping the reality of losing both breasts and getting "dummy" ones. Don't get me wrong I am very blessed and grateful for this gift and have never and will never ever blame you for this I thank you, however, it is getting overwhelming and I find myself wondering if you would have done the same if you had had the chance and knowledge that I have. I picked silicone implants they look much better made and feel better but I may need tissue expanders to help stretch muscle to fit an implant my size. We told the kids tonight too. I wanted them to know so they didn't worry, we didn't make it as serious as it is. I was worried Emily may ask if she would get sick boobies but she didn't so I am glad. I just wanted them to know what to expect to see over next week. We joked about how big I would be! Emily liked that!

ॐ⸱ॐ   ॐ⸱ॐ   ॐ⸱ॐ

Dad Tammy and Simone all want to be there I would really prefer them not to be its hard enough to go through without an audience. Now I know how you felt and I am sorry if I was ever there at the hospital when you really didn't want me there. I understand it's hard enough to keep it together for yourself let alone an audience of loved ones. But as I did with you, they have a need to be there for me. Dad for his daughter, because my mom who should be there can't be and Tammy as my sister, huge supporter, and my friend Simone, she seems the most upset by this and worried. I hope she will see it is all ok. I think she is in shock of what is happening.

Someone admired your ring today on my finger, and every time someone does I want to think it's your way of letting me know you are with me always.

I pray my kids don't miss and hurt as much as I miss and ache for you when I am gone. It is so painful but I don't want the pain to stop because I fear I will forget you and I don't want to, the pain keeps you fresh — if that makes any sense at all.

The loss and ache deep down in my gut is awful it's almost been a year and every time I see your picture I cry.

I saw the bench Dad made in your memory, you would like it Mom. And there will be a dedication plate on it saying "Come sit a while" dedicated to the memory of Diane M. Hunt. He is so proud of it. He seems happy and busy with friends and I would rather that than worrying about him being alone all the time and lonely. I am amazed everyday at how strong he had been in his loss. Why am I not? You were his family, I have my family, why do I feel more affected? I can only guess it's because of what I will go through this next year to eradicate the potential of cancer from my body and generations to come with the knowledge of BRCA1 you gave us. Friday I go for pre op. Monday is go day. I will write you soon after ok. I know you will be there with me and I pray to see you in my deep anesthetic sleep! Hint hint!

I love you so much,
Tracy XO

Journal Excerpt: March 3, 2007

Hi Mom. Well one more day till my surgery and I am still nervous I don't know exactly why I was feeling good about it again till my pre op appt on Friday. Just really anxious about the afterwards. The pain, the recovery. I want to get back to me (normal) as quickly as possible. I know, trust me I will take care of myself and rest and will do all the proper foods and exercises because I really want to be good for the move. I know you will be there with me. Went to the Falls today, wanted the kids to have a nice weekend before I am off for a bit. We took Jeanette, she hasn't been in a long time, so it was nice for her. She is doing a scrapbook for the kids of today — so nice. Also bought me some nice pj's for when I come home. She has been very supportive. She is picking up the kids on Monday after school for us. I will be home Tuesday morning. Its weird my breasts will be gone but I am thankful that chemo doesn't have to follow and my journey ends here, almost.

I see your struggle now differently, more personally mom. You were so brave and strong — all the drains, surgeries, chemos, drugs, needles, I can't believe it. Some say I am strong and brave, but I am actually chicken. I am not strong enough to face any future of cancer again, so this is a given, a have to. I am grateful, and yes, could have just had yearly MRIs but I am your daughter and know if I keep my breasts and ovaries.....I can't.

I will touch base with you next week verbally, will be looking for you as I sleep on Monday so I hope you do come to see me.

Love you so much,
Tracy tree XO

Journal Excerpt: March 5, 2007

Well they cancelled my surgery at the last minute. What an emotional mental ride I have been on. Now I have to go in on Friday. There was an emergency that took precedence. Man, all the planning prep for the kids, psyching myself up, I came home and just cried and slept! Now I have to go through it all over again. I was calm today too. I was ready. Anyway wanted you to know about the change I am sure you already did! So I will see you Friday now.

Love you Mom, see you Friday.

Tracy xo

Journal Excerpt: March 15, 2007

Hi Mom. Well almost 1 week after surgery, to sore to write till today. It makes me very sad and lonely that you aren't here and no one I know can relate to what I am going through. I looked yesterday for the first time and just sobbed. I look like a horrible dismembered woman. I know and try to think this isn't how they will look in 6 months-1 yr but right now it's awful I wasn't prepared and am glad I chose reconstruction now that I see.

I have tissue expanders in as the implants I chose were too small! Funny eh! They took 600 cc's from each breast and implants were 470 cc. so all went well and I will be pumped up weekly and in 6 months have permanent implants to replace the expanders. I am feeling better today each day is getting better, less pain, more movement. My left side has a little more fluid and is red around the scarring so I will keep an eye on it I have been massaging it to help fluid disperse. Had drains removed this morning and first shower later on. That was hard again as I saw my complete distorted body. I just keep telling myself I am in extreme makeover! I better have nice ones!!!

I try to focus on the move soon too I am excited for that. I have been alone most of the time- all day- like you used to be and it gets very lonely. Yesterday I barely got out of bed all day very depressed. I worry about the kids, if this will have a long term effect on them, try to be positive around them, but also honest of how I am feeling they went to camp and daycare out early home late, so it's been a long week for them and very out of routine.

I just want to get back to myself you know. Back to work back to routines and able to pack etc. I will wait though and have done NOTHING since I got home. Rick has been good with everything I haven't shown him as I don't want him to see and have that vision in his head. I want him to remember me as I was. He said it doesn't bother him, he wants me healthy and for a long time. He is very loving and supportive and hasn't made me feel less of a woman.

He says he will have a wife with big firm boobs and no periods! Every man's dream!!

I have planned to leave my shirt on even during sex, whenever that will be, I know that he feels differently than me, but as it was for me, it is different when you see it.

Getting tired will talk later.

Love Tracy

ABOUT MY MASTECTOMY

Honestly, it was a painful recovery, emotionally, physically and mentally. I was back to work in three weeks, I had to. It was either sit home, lonely or get out and live. I still remember the first question my surgeon asked me the next day after the surgery when she came to see me was "do you have any regrets." I said "no."

She said if I did, they could arrange counseling for me, as many women do have an understandably difficult time afterwards.

I never regretted my decision, but did have to live in my now: the pain, no breasts, or the implants as I wanted. Now I had to go through expansion, a step I didn't plan for.

My advice to any woman making this decision: plan something, say six to eight weeks from the surgery that will give you something to look forward to and focus you on something positive.

Many thought I was nuts to have my moving date seven weeks from my surgery, but I needed it to be that way. This was a dream I had had for a long time, and it was the right timing for me.

Through my recovery and the seven weeks to our move, each day I did a little packing, bit by bit (we didn't have that much honestly). I believe moving into my new home was well overshadowing the loss of my breasts and the physical recovery I had to do.

I didn't know it, but breast tissue is attached to the pectoral muscles, so I had no use of my arms when I came out of surgery, and for a couple weeks, had to do special exercises to get them working again! I think this was the only side effect I wasn't expecting. There were no other complications. My surgeon was the best, very clean, very caring. I knew I was in good hands in this journey.

But it had only just begun. Little did I know, what I thought would be a quick six-month turnaround, has now been over a year. I had one expander leak, so it needed to be replaced nine weeks later. I did that under a local anesthetic. I didn't want to go under again as I had a very rough time coming out. I found out I had allergy to morphine! So I was in and out, and home and back to work in a week after that procedure. Then, with summer, delays happened with vacations. And I needed to be 600cc's. I didn't want to be less. They do 60cc a week in each expander; they insert a needle into a port in my chest that goes into the expander and closes when the needle is pulled out (like filling up a basketball). It didn't hurt as I had no nerves there, so everything was and will remain forever, along that incision line, numb to touch. So, even when I get nipples, they will only be for cosmetic purposes. They won't have any feeling. But I am not Barbie, so don't want to anatomically look like her. I want my nips! So with 60cc/week, that worked out to 10 weeks…but….

I didn't want to do my surgery in my business 4th quarter, so I opted to put it off till spring. Then another incentive came; a trip to Barbados. I had to win that, man. God, everyone knew I could use that trip!!!

During all this, my periods were getting worse, something I didn't pay much attention to as had so much other going on. But they got worse, heavy, clotty, painful, very painful, and they started and never stopped!! So I made the decision to have the oopherectomy and implant exchange together in February, however, no such luck. For whatever reason, they couldn't do both together, so I had my oopherectomy on February 20, 2008, and was back and earned that trip to Barbados!!!!

I was back from my beautiful trip to Barbados on April 23, and had my implant exchange on May 1! And, they are beautiful! I did this surgery under a local with some sedation as well, was home same day, and back to work in a week!

Because I wasn't a top 20 manager the year before as I had hoped to be, I had to do it this year. I wanted to move up in the company, and they wanted me to as well, however, I needed that credibility. So I am going to do it this year, I am ready to move on, move forward, and move up! Remember, you need something else to focus on, to get you through something like this. Otherwise you stay in it, and it gets harder and harder to get out of it. I allowed myself to feel it, the sadness, the pain, but then I moved off it, and moved forward. I looked to what was ahead, and that is what got me back to work quicker, I am healthy and never compromised my health, but didn't stay in that place that would only bring me down. That wasn't my mother; it wasn't me. I told her I would make her proud. I saw how she fought and lived, and I was going to do the same. There was no time for any other choice. Ever.

ॐ✞ॐ ॐ✞ॐ ॐ✞ॐ

My next step is my nipples. The icing on the cake, the mustard on the hot dog, the salt on the margarita!   And they will be beautiful too, my twins, my non-cancer-causing twins.

Journal Excerpt: March 24, 2007

Well it's my first birthday without your morning "happy birthday song" musical call. I used to expect it every year. You were always the first to call with Dad. I really missed it this morning, as I received no calls at all.

Dad gave me a very nice card and money yesterday. He came by and we took him through the new house. I am getting anxious to move now! So many plans! You would love it and would be very proud Mom.

Simone came and visited took her to see your resting place. I couldn't help but cry as I always do. I still can't believe I have made it this long and been through so much without you here these past 10 months.

I wondered while I was there what you would have advised me to do. I think you would have not advised this, but would have supported me. Know your death had a reason in, your death you brought me and Emily life! The greatest gift of all. Your death was not for nothing it had purpose, you kept wondering why you? And this was why Mom, to save me, your first born from battling the same war as you.

I will always be grateful. I am still wondering why you haven't come to comfort me. I have needed you more than anyone. Maybe you are in heaven now.

I am doing much better mentally and emotionally, physically still need to catch up, still tire quickly.

Gonna head downstairs now, kids have a gift for me.

Love your "Tracy tree" now 36!

XOXOX

Journal Excerpt: April 2, 2007

Hey Mom. I started back to work today. Also starting to feel like I am coming down with something. Any way, thinking about you a lot lately. I am starting to feel melancholy as we are approaching the 1 year anniversary of your death. I can't believe how this year has flown by. There has not been ONE day that I haven't thought about you missed you wished you were here. I know you know. I am trying to remember last year, last Easter and I can't. Did I have Easter? Did Tammy? What were you like? I hate that I cannot remember. What I hate even more is soon I won't be able to think "last year when mom was here".

෨ঔ ෨ঔ ෨ঔ

Now I wonder what this next year holds for Dad now that his year of mourning is over. Will he get together with anyone? I am crying for you over you tonight, as if you died today. As I was crying and looking at the picture of you and me and a teardrop fell on the picture of you and smeared—I am so upset, it erased part of your skin and hair DAMN IT! I can't get another one like it DAMN IT. What picture does that? I have never had that happen. I am really upset now. It is the pik of you and I that I have stared at, and cried to since the day you gave it to me. Every time you deteriorated I would hold that picture, and every time since, and this is weird, the frame you chose, the pink marble, is the same color stone we picked for your pillow stone at your resting place!

That pik has been a constant in my life in your absence. A security blanket for me and now I ruined it. DAMN IT.

God Mom, why haven't you come to see me in my dreams? You know I need you please please I need you Mom. This has been difficult without you. I knew the day the Dr said you had BRCA1 I knew I had it too that is why I left and cried in the bathroom and Dad had to come and get me, I knew it in my gut but didn't want you to know that. I think you knew too. I wished we had talked about it more before you died. We never discussed it except for you telling me they'd be in touch from McMaster. Why didn't we ever talk about it, did you talk about it with dad?

Love you
Tracy xo

Journal Excerpt: April 12, 2007

Hi Mom. Today I had my first fill up went well. I felt a little faint and queezy after but recovered quickly there was no pain.

Guess what?! Avon is donating $5000 to the BGH! Because of me!! My tulip planting there in the fall put them on the list of community donations Avon was going to give across Canada!

I present a check to them in May. Dad was here tonight, said the pink tulips are coming up at your site. I can't wait to see them. 18 days till we move! I can't wait mom. We are having a garage sale this weekend to get rid of stuff and make some money...

I cried for you today after I had my needle. I thought about all the needles you had with your drainings and chemos how you must have felt but hid from us. You were so strong mom. People say I am but I don't see it, I guess cause they don't see my tears and weak moments I guess you had yours too, you must have but you never let us see it either. Sometimes I wish you would have. Emily wanted to see my breasts tonight, so I showed her. She asked a few more questions, but still hasn't linked it to her, I am grateful I am not ready to answer that. I would probably say we don't need to worry about that right now.

She wanted to see where they put the needle in my expander. I believe because her and Jack have known and seen, they have handled it better, rather than having to imagine the worst they can see it and ask all the questions they want. I was tired today also I have strep throat so I have taken it easy today. When your year anniversary comes up we are going to your grave and Rick will play Amazing Grace on his bagpipes and then we will lay flowers and go to our house for food.

I cant wait to move in, I am still nervous! I hope it all goes smooth and we get the keys first thing! Take care of that eh!

Love you Mom, come see me ok.

Tracy

Journal Excerpt: May 1, 2007

Hey Mom. So sorry haven't written in awhile so busy moving! Well, we are officially in! and home owners again Mom. I got the key at 130pm April 30 and I cried for you all the way to the new house, with that key in my hand. I went to the cemetery to see you this morning — the tulips are coming up!

The house is beautiful and perfect and bigger than we have ever had before. You would be proud I wish you were here Mom. More good news — The Expositor wants to do a Mother's day piece on my story! Can you believe it Mom! They feel it is a great inspiring story, it combines the donation from Avon to the BGH and my story about a Mom, for Mother's day.

We are 10 days away from the 1 year mark. I have really really ached for you today. Maybe because so physically and mentally and emotionally tired. I am whipped, what a month!

Out of regular routine too, I have hardly eaten the past couple days so busy. House is all set up except for living room, we are getting new furniture for it. We have been here for 1 day but look like we have been here for months! Piks up and all! But you know me, I am a master packer and unpacker and make any place I am in, home asap!

All family helped, Mike and Diane came down from Kingston and stayed to help, even though they were supposed to be back that night, I am so appreciative.

Anyway, gonna go wind down and watch move with Rick in our new basement!!! I love you and we did it Mom!!

Dreams do come true!

Xox Tracy

Journal Excerpt: May 11, 2007

1 YEAR ANNIVERSARY

Hi Mom. It was a hard day to concentrate today. I kept remembering the events from a year ago today. I woke up the same time when Tammy called me a year ago saying you had stopped breathing and EMS was at the house. It echoes in my head. I miss you.

Today we all went to your grave and laid pink flowers and talked about and cried about how we made it a year without you and how we wish we didn't have to. Rick played Amazing Grace on his bagpipes, same as John did the day you were buried (–can you believe Rick plays them now!!) you would be laughing and coughing…

We came back and had supper here. Dad was weepy today. I think it is hitting him as he is now missing Diane, his healthy wife, not the sick one he cared for as a patient. Now we start another year. But you are always here very very close to me Mom. I did the event at the hospital yesterday where I presented the check from Avon. The tulips look good and they took my pik and will be in the paper they feel my story will inspire others.

A whole year later. I never imagined any of this good would come from your illness and death. But so much has mom, so much has.

I love you thank you for doing that test.

Love Tracy xox

Journal Excerpt: May 14, 2007

Mothers day

Happy Mother's day Mom. Dad did a beautiful BBQ at his house for me Tammy and Nan. He had Uncle Doug and Aunt Katie and Uncle John and Ricks' Mom there too. He set the backyard up beautifully kids had a great time too. Katie painted their faces, they love that! It was a really nice day. I love Dad for doing it. Kept my mind somewhat off the fact that you were the one mother missing. But you were in all our thoughts. I know that.

My story- our story- was in the paper yesterday! A full page!!! You'd be very proud! I don't know if there are any copies left for anyone between us all buying them up!!! Dad was very weepy and proud of me too, I think he is in shock of all I have done and that I went public! You know how private he is...

Love ya Mom.

Tracy xox

Journal Excerpt: May 24, 2007

Mom I can't believe it one of my implants ruptured and has gone flat. My left one. They have to get me in asap to replace it. I have opted to have the permanent implants put in as I can't go through anymore. I want this to be the final stage of this breast thing. I wish you were here Mom why is this happening to me. I have been so good so brave so smart about all of this — now this happens.

I think it was punctured at my last fill, I have done nothing to cause this. The nurse said was a freak thing and some are defective. Work is going so well I am doing well, now this happens. They are calling this afternoon to tell me surgery date. Will keep you posted. As you always you to say!

Love u
Tracy xo

Journal Excerpt: June 1, 2007

Hi Mom. Jun 11 is my surgery day, they couldn't get me in any sooner, so I am currently lopsided! I hate having this useless foreign thing in me.

I want to do it with just a local anesthetic like you did for your mastectomy. I will recover quicker and feel better. I hope they will do it that way for me. I am ok for now. Wish this didn't happen but everything happens for a reason right. Hope to only be off 1 week. Family is all well. Dad is busy at work don't see much of him. We all went to Tammy's in laws cottage last weekend, Dad took his camper, the kids had fun. It's boat season so he will be going out on his boat a lot I think.

Anyway heading to bed. Been busy week. So tired.

Love you mom, where are you? Come see me please been thinking of contacting that psychic I saw in Vegas...

Love Tracy xox

Journal Excerpt: June 6, 2007

Went to doctors today. I am feeling very sad and angry and confused. The doctor doesn't want to do implants for medical and personal reasons. Scar could open and expose implant as skin/muscle not totally stretch, and she is concerned I am making wrong decision because of my upset of another surgery she believes I will be unhappy in the long run with much smaller breasts as I was adamant about retuning to my size from beginning until this hiccup in my road.

She said would only delay things for month or so but would be worth it. Rick agreed, he has said that since I made the decision. So I am listening to her and him as I can't make it alone and am very emotional right now and don't want to make wrong decision. But I really do want this to be done Mom. I am sure you felt and said that to yourself many times on your journey, but you didn't give up, you did what it took and always took Drs advice so today I did the same. I worry about the interruptions it is causing in my life and career, silly I know but I didn't think it would be this much. I hope I have honored your memory this past year in the things I have done and decisions I have made. This journal is so cathartic for me I really feel connected to you when I write in it, like you can actually read and hear it!

I was in a store yesterday, and swear you were there as I walked down one isle and the same version of "Danny Boy" that we had at your funeral was playing and the next isle I walked down they were playing Amazing Grace, like John did at your funeral on the bagpipes. Was this coincidence? They were those CD players you can play out certain songs before you buy, but the one CD was songs of nature, no Danny boy, and the other wasn't a bagpipe collection, that was very very weird! Was it you letting me know you were there? And you were with me? I am wanting to believe it was! Mom today I need you. I feel tired and weak from putting on this brave front for everyone and just want to crawl away most days. Is this how you felt a lot? You were so brave as well, it must have tired you as I know it wasn't easy for you.

I love you and respect you and admire you. I am so blessed to be Diane Margaret Hunt's daughter.

Love Tracy tree xoxox

Journal Excerpt: June 12, 2007

Well home after surgery. I was home yesterday but too tired to write. Did exchange under a local and I was awake for surgery but I didn't feel a thing. Painful today but felt much better than I did after surgery in March.

They filled it to 250cc, so only 2 fills away from my right one. Only taking Advil and Gravol very nauseated. Wish you were here. Miss you. Wearing your coral track jacket so you are around me, like hugging me. Gonna go to sleep now very tired.

Love ya Mom

Journal Excerpt: July 8, 2007

Hey Mom

Was looking back in my journal and I realized I never shared with you the impact our story had on some women. I received calls from the newspaper article they did on me for Mother's day. Some calls came a week to 2 weeks after and couple phoned today.

These women all had breast cancer and were clear but had daughters and wanted more info on how to get testing. They weren't aware of it and needed to know where to start. This is why I decided to go public to begin with. It made our journey meaningful because we have now given power, empowered other women in similar situations to get answers and knowledge they need to pro act and possibly save their daughters from this disease. I am thankful you took the test part of me still wishes you were here physically with me but you were very private and I don't think you would have wanted to go public. These women said I was strong and brave and wise. And they wished me luck on my continued journey.

They also said it made them realize that peace of mind was worth more than 2 mounds of flesh and tissue on their chest, as I had said they are "just boobs" in the article, they said others who read it said I struck a nerve with that and it caused a realization. Ricks aunt sent me a beautiful card, offering her support and admiration of the love I had for my family to do what I did. I am going to put that card and the paper article in this journal as well. You would be proud of me mom. I am doing well. Had a fill last week and then again this Friday. They are "growing" nicely!

Kids are at camp this week. They love it.

Talk later

Love Tracy xox

Journal Excerpt: August 4, 2007

Hey Mom

Thinking of you today. We went up to Barrie for a drive to see our old place and take kids to "our" beach for a swim.

Floods of memories of you came back. Us waiting on the beach for Dad and Rick to come around the bend in the boat to pick us up, canoeing along the shoreline, looking into people's backyards and how the rich lived! You and Dad coming to stay on weekends at "your cottage' breaky in the morning at the hummingbird and then to Top Dollar to get Emily a treat.

You loved that little house. It was like your cottage, like you called it! And we loved having you very much. The house looks good our front garden is now grass, they sodded it in and the pine tree is healthy and big as are the birch trees we replanted. Street same, still gravel and major potholes! Had some regrets about selling it. Rick still regrets us not keeping it and renting it out, but he fails to remember our financial position at the time, we needed to sell it to move home we couldn't afford to rent it. I wish we could've though.

I reminded him that money allowed him to start on his own, it funded his business and us for that first year, and to pay off debts. He thinks we would have been fine but I know we wouldn't have. I regret leaving the atmosphere, the relaxed living but since you are gone it wouldn't have been the same anyway and would have been much too small for us now, we outgrew that home the moment we had Jack anyway.

It was nice to go back, to connect with lost memories. But it also reminded me of the tough time we had up there alone. Maybe one day we will head back there. It isn't like it was anyway, it is building up so much now, it's like a city, not cottage country anymore. You wouldn't believe all the houses there now!

We think we will take our bikes up there next time and go biking around our old tracks and maybe take canoe. Maybe Dad will come. Maybe not. He wouldn't go to the Falls with us, said reminded him too much of you.

Nothing else to report.

I love you

Tracy xox

Journal Excerpt: August 28, 2007

Happy anniversary Mom.

You and Dad would have been married 37 years today. I took pink tulips to your gravesite, felt compelled to. Went to see Dad tonite with kids and Tammy went with kids to acknowledge the day for Dad. We got him a gift card and Tammy got him a beautiful card and going forward, this will be our "family anniversary" as it is the day we became a family. I really like that idea. Dad not only made his commitment to you but to us too.

We are going up to the cottage in Sauble this weekend with dad he is looking forward to it and we always go with him the first weekend. I mean we always did with you and him. Was missing you today I cried for you. Kids are getting excited for school. Got all the kids school supplies, took me back to when you used to get ours from Canadian tire, we could load up the cart with whatever we wanted, we loved that day!!! And you would let us play with them outside, you never made us pack them away and not let us use them. we would sharpen all of our pencil crayons and play school for hours...(maybe that is why you did it, to keep us out of your hair??)

We always got a new outfit for school too! I let Emily and Jack do the same and they model their clothes for Daddy, Jack not so much!

My work conference went well, always enjoy going. I can't believe it was a year ago I got my results, now here I am a year later, still don't have my implants and no oopherectomy done yet, longer road than I anticipated.

It's still hard for me to visit Dad at the house. I always think of you. I rarely go there, he usually comes here.

Love you Mom xox

Tracy

Journal Excerpt: October 6, 2007

Happy Thanksgiving Mom. I haven't written in awhile, almost a month and I can feel when I haven't. I don't feel right, guilty kind of. I finished my last fill, I am now 660cc which is like having a bag of milk on each breast they say!

Finding a little strain in breathing and my left breast aches, bruised feeling underarm area and where the port is but it will go away. Feel like have elephants sitting on my chest like after my mastectomy surgery.

They look pretty real and good to me. A full C size, very very hard though like I am engorged!

I go back in 4 mths then have surgery in about 5 mths along with my oopherectomy. After that few months later will have nipples tattooed and then I am complete!

Won't have to worry about cancer there or wear a bra or pad again! Thank you!!

Some days are still tough though. I know there are foreign objects in my body but cancer probably felt that way to you right?

I have wished for you lately cried for you lately I still miss you terrible.

I am doing big turkey this year again, will have 22 here tomorrow, yes I am crazy.

Work is going good, I hope to go to Barbados in April. Kids are doing well, in hockey and figure skating and Emily getting A's in her new school. Rick and I are good.

I wish I could feel your hugs again. They live still strong in my memory. I can't believe this is our second Thanksgiving without you. This year I am thankful I made it through my surgery well and I am almost done.

Love Trac xox

Journal Excerpt: December 3, 2007

Hey Mom. Need you today. Went for appt with doctor doing my oopherectomy. I told her of the troubles I have been having and the changes and she was concerned so did a biopsy right in her office, symptoms of cervical cancer. She will call in a week with the results. She said they need to do it before surgery to confirm so they get no surprises in operating room.

I have asked to have surgery Feb 15 as that is when the incentive for Barbados ends I know Mom, but I am doing it earlier than I planned to, I was going to wait until the summer, but I need it done now. I will be recouped and ready for the trip on Apr 19 this way.

I really want to get promoted too, so I need to earn these incentives. Rick is behind me all the way. He is a good father and husband, I am very lucky (most days!).

Take care, I hope I don't have cancer, I have too much to accomplish I don't have time for it, to be honest.

All will be ok.

Love you

Tracy xox

Journal Excerpt: December 10, 2007

Biopsy negative, all is good, probably endometriosis, so glad to be getting this procedure done.

Love ya, Tracy xo

Journal Excerpt: January 1, 2008

Well another year gone by and another to go through without you. Christmas was good. We got a DVD from Dads friend of you at one of their Christmas events. I haven't had the heart to watch it yet. I haven't watched you on any DVD I have of you since Emily's birthday last year. It's too hard.

Everyone is well. I go for my surgery on Feb 20 for the oopherectomy.

Love you

Tracy xox

Journal Excerpt: February 17, 2008

Hi Mom

Had Dad over tonight for supper. He seemed agitated. Said he was painting the house to sell it. Said he wants to move up north to get a log cabin on the lake! Retire early and live off the interest. I had to go upstairs cause I started to cry…it upset me. Just the matter of fact way he said it. I guess I am angry and sad, I moved out here and now he wants to move away, I don't want him to move away, or sell the house. I don't know if he was trying to get a rise out of me, to see my reaction, why would he do that just days before my surgery? How could he cope with no family around for him. He said we could come up in the summer for a couple of weeks. I asked if he'd been looking and he said no but someone he knew did it and he wanted to. I could hear you tonite, saying "oh tom"! He must be lonely Mom. I don't know what to do for him. I invited him tonite I haven't had him over in awhile; he bought me lovely Valentine's card and chocolates, a beautiful card, it said

> *Dear daughter*
> *This little valentine comes from the heart for once upon a time, when you were my funny peanut butter and jelly face the angel girl I fell in love with who I could hold and hug forever. You're my beautiful daughter wise beyond your years worrying me one day and inspiring me the next. Today and always I'm so proud of you (he underlined proud) and I love you with all my heart.*
> *Love Dad*

Rick said not to pay attention to him about selling the house, not to take it too serious. I know Dad is not a creature of change, but a creature of habit. He won't initiate change, but will change only if it is inflicted upon him.

I miss you badly at these times Mom, none of these conversations would be happening if you were still here.

I am anxious to get this surgery done, not so much nervous. It brings me 1 step closer to ending this journey. And it has been a long road. I am glad I have kept this journal, for 2 years in May! It has truly helped me and kept me close to you.

Love your
Tracy tree
xox

Journal Excerpt: February 19, 2008

Be with me tomorrow Mom. My last major surgery on this journey to cancer prevention in my family.

Love you thank you. Will be ok.

Tracy xo

Journal Excerpt: February 24, 2008

Hi Mom. Well 4 days post surgery. It went very well. And I am doing well. Was home the same day again!!! I amaze the nurses!

Pretty sore up till today moving a little better no pain except for when I have to go number 2, bowels working ok they finally started today and no problems with my plumbing!

Tummy is swollen but that will go down and only 4 small incisions! One is in the belly button so not even noticeable, amazing! They took ovaries, tubes through incision and cervix and then vacuumed uterus through my vagina, unbelievable. The bleeding has stopped. Never again! Yay!

I am in good spirits not like after the mastectomy, that was tough, physically, emotionally, this one was welcomed!

Now I will be on calcium daily to prevent early onset of osteoporosis (as I am 20 years ahead of menopause so 20 years ahead for osteo as well). I go see the doctor in 1 month.

Back to work March 5 then off again for March break with the kids. Its been tough having Rick do everything again, I remember you needing us and can now relate again. I only have to give up a few days of not doing anything, you did it for a year, almost. Mom, if I ever made you feel like you were putting me out I so apologize, but now, know I am ok, I will be ok. No more breast or ovarian cancer in this family. I have also vowed to stop being a social smoker. It makes no sense, absolute stupidity for me to continue after what I have endured to prevent getting it. I am smart, not stupid, so know that. Emily made me a beautiful card, on the front it said "super girl, supergirl" inside she wrote

Dear mom
I hope you feel better soon and I wrote you a
poem. Please read it.

Operations are painful
And when you are lonely
People come and come
To give you flowers cards and other things to
And they wish to you
And say I hope you feel better soon.
Love Emily Jack Daddy Spanky and Max.
On the other fold she wrote
We love you
Hope you feel better soon.
Oxoxoxoxoxxooxoxoxoxxoxo
Xoxoxoxoxoxooxoxoxoxoxox
Roses are red
Violets are blue
Nothing is better
Without you!

I will cherish it and keep it always!

Love you
Tracy xox

Journal Excerpt: March 10, 2008

Hey Mom. I earned the trip to Barbados!!!!! Finally I did it!!! Don't really care about going just wanted to win it!

It is from Apr 19-23. I already wrote list of what I need to take and do before I go!

I started spotting again and got a urinary tract infection. They say this is all normal.

I am hot flashing big time! More so at night in bed. Disturbs my sleep and last few days felt grouchy and tired!

I see the doctor on Mar 27 so will talk then about solutions. Also have to start calcium and vitamin D, and weight training, they all help prevent osteoporosis.

My birthday is coming up, Easter is same weekend this year. We are doing Easter dinner here, I know I am crazy again!

∿∿   ∿∿   ∿∿

I can't believe we are coming up to 2 years without you. I can't believe I have 2 years worth of feelings in here. I am glad I have, it has helped me I believe get through all I have had to , to put my thoughts my true thoughts down to you my Mom and for me you can really only move on from honesty to your true destination, right.

I am content with my job, my house, we want to buy income properties down the road, and I still want that hardtop tent trailer too, and Disney, always Disney!

Love ya
Tracy xo

Journal Excerpt: March 17, 2008

Hi Mom. I dreamt of you last night. I was walking home from a restaurant after working with some managers to your home down Glenwood and I saw you and Dad sitting together on the porch. I couldn't believe it!

In my dream though, you and Dad had separated and you came back after a long vacation to visit Dad and when I saw you I cried and cried. And said I had dreams you died and to see you again was unbelievable. You hugged me, you looked great, I remember you were wearing a nice red sweater and nice necklace and chocolate brown shirt over it and pants. You truly looked amazing. Your hair was red and short. Then....I woke up and cried. You had also brought lots of Christmas presents you said you made a mistake calling Tammy so much while you were on vacation cause you shopped for everybody! I followed Dad to the garage to help him put some of the presents away and a cat came down from the attic. As I was in the garage, I thought, what am I doing, I need to go hug mom and kiss her. I came back to you and hugged you so tight. Very weird how I remember the whole dream with clarity also the reason I left the restaurant and walked so fast home was because I felt creeped out by one guy who kept touching me as he walked by me!

ॐ✧ ॐ✧ ॐ✧

I will never forget how I felt when I saw you on the porch with Dad, it is truly how I would feel if I ever did see you again. Overwhelmed, shocked, disbelief, soooo happy, emotional, but in my dream you weren't dead, just back from a separation with Dad.

Thank you for hugging me, I love you Mom and I miss you immensely. That dream teased me, I hate that I woke up.

Love

Tracy xox

Journal Excerpt: April 25, 2008

Hi Mom. Well what an amazing trip I had to Barbados!!
I know you were there with me. I went snorkeling and saw shipwrecks, and sea turtles and amazing fish. I toured the island, drank a bit, had some great laughs and relaxed! I am so glad I achieved it.

I feel guilty I didn't really miss home. Is that bad? I didn't miss work or chores or arguments.

I really needed that trip now I see why people spend money to go on tropical vacations, I have been bitten by the bug!

Surgery is next week, final one!

Next on my list...lose 30 lbs, I have gained weight this past year, I really have to lose it and get toned.

ॐ৵ৎ   ॐ৵ৎ   ॐ৵ৎ

Some sad news, a neighbor of yours who was good to you when you were ill has been diagnosed with breast cancer. Dad heard from her husband the other day.

I will send her a card to let her know I am thinking of her. This disease is horrible. Will we ever stop it?

ॐ৵ৎ   ॐ৵ৎ   ॐ৵ৎ

Dad has been out riding his motorcycle, he loves it! He feels very badly for our friend, part of him is reluctant to get involved again with someone because he fears he will have to go through it again, I told him he can't not fall in love again because he is afraid they will die. He said he is afraid of the cancer.

I talked about you on my trip. I miss you dearly can't believe 2 years almost.

Dad is having mother's day again this year. Will be hard this year though as it falls on your 2 year anniversary, May 11.

I lost you too soon mom. I really really did. Does God know he made a mistake and took the wrong person at the wrong time?

Love you so much

Tracy xo

Journal Excerpt: April 29, 2008

Hi Mom. 2 days till my permanent boobs! Tammy wants to come and I told her it would be ok. I am not nervous glad to be done this chapter in my life.

Dad and Tammy bought me an ottoman for the living room as a "your finally done" gift!! So nice of them!

And then today Tammy and I went and split on a patio set for Dad, he has wanted one, and he has been amazing, we took it to his house and he was in shock!!

He was pleasantly surprised.

I keep thinking of telling my story, but it's not a unique one I don't think. I am not the only woman been diagnosed BRCA1 positive. Who would read my story? Why do I want to share this story?

Rick reminded me of my paper article a year ago, and how it impacted many and how I got calls, he said, there are many books out there, on the same subject, and he encouraged me to do it.

I want to make it a motivational, inspiring book. All I know is in my gut, my story needs to be told how attitude truly can open your mind and heart and allow you to get through anything and come out the other side with more hope than you had going in.

Will keep you posted!

Love ya

Tracy xo

Journal Excerpt: May 3, 2008

Hey Mom. Well had surgery May 1, couldn't write till now. Been in bed, last 2 days more pain that I anticipated actually felt like I had the mastectomy again! Was sick last night, the first night, Rick said combo of the drugs, the anxiety the surgery itself takes a toll, but I am good now.

I did it all with a local and some sedation! I hope when the bandages come off they look good! They don't seem big, course all the bandages don't help me see them really. I am glad to be done! I was in and out within 4 hrs!! I thought I would be off 1 week only but now it's looking like 2 weeks from what Doctor said.

Kids are good.

Mom. I am done. Wish you were here with me. I know you would have been at the hospital throughout this past year.

I have had lots of support and well wishers!

Gonna go rest some more, very tired.

Love you mom, we are done!!!

Tracy xox

THE JOURNEY'S ENDING

The end of this long chapter in my life presented me with an overwhelming feeling to share it. What better than a book? I had been writing it without knowing it for the last two years, an idea of writing that started the day my mom died. What better way to symbolize my victory, my journey's end, than to bring it all together and give other women this knowledge that could save their lives.

After all, the written word is every person's opportunity to live forever. And, really, isn't this what we all want? Isn't it why we fight these fights, these battles, with courage and hope of victory, and to look back at the end of a hardship or disease and see all the footprints in our sand?

I did pre-survive breast and ovarian cancer. I am a pre-survivor. I did make it through, and I did look back, and to my comfort, I saw many, many footprints in my sand.

And, thank you to every set of them: the doctors and nurses, my work family, my friends, but most of all to my family, my husband, Richard, my children Emily and Jack, my dad, Tom, my sister, Tammy. Thank you, for their unwaivering, unquestioning love and support. Always.

Mom left us a stronger, more loving, more courageous family. Her dream came true. We are her legacy that allows her to live on forever.

I love you all.

A LETTER TO MY HUSBAND

Where to start? This is the hardest part of this book, trying to get down in words the magnitude of my love and respect for you. How do you tell the one person you love most in this world what they have done for you? I knew from the moment I saw you that August, 18 years ago, that we would be together forever.

Through our time together, you have loved me, supported me, challenged me, angered me, and understood my ambitious quest to want more in life, as I did you. I can't tell you enough how important you were to me through these past couple of years.

From the moment we heard mom was sick, you never said no to me about anything. You agreed to sell the house, even though I know you didn't want to, loved the kids more for me when I was dealing with my grief, and at times gave up what you wanted to carry me through this time when you knew I just couldn't handle one more thing. You sacrificed many things, too, and lost big these past couple of years, in your personal quests for your dreams. We are not done, yet. You are the father to our kids, as my dad was to me. Although you didn't have a father figure in your life, you just know how to be a great dad, never question that. You were with me from the first blood test to the diagnoses, and you wanted me to do whatever it took to live, never once waivering.

You never made me feel less than a woman when I lost my breasts. When I cried about it, you were there, always the light of reason and constant love and strength. You were there for the kids; you kept life going for them when I couldn't. You kept me laughing, yelling, living, and dreaming.

You have supported my ambition with my career always. You have loved me through the loss of my mom, and you have carried me through some of the most important decisions about my life.

You are my best friend. I love you so much more than I ever imagined a person could love. You gave me two beautiful children, and a life that feels protected and sacred. That is truly all a woman can ask for.

I Love You.

Tracy

A LETTER TO MY DAD

Dad,

Every time I think of you, tears come to my eyes. Not because I am sad for you but because I get overwhelmed at the love I feel for you, and the admiration I have for you.

You were always there, growing up. You were always home; you were always involved in our lives. You were the neighborhood dad who made cool things for everyone. If one of our neighborhood friends saw something you made us and liked it, you made them one to. Whether it was making stilts, track equipment in the backyard, or chasing us to let us know we could never out-run our "old man." You were a constant of light in my and Tammy's life.

Whatever we needed, you provided. We didn't have the name brand stuff or the best of anything, but looking back, all I remember is having dinner together every night, but not eating till mom heard all about your day! She lived through you and your social circle!

You were never out with the guys; we were your guys. You never made us feel we were bothering or interrupting you or that your time was more valuable elsewhere. You never yelled at us. You treated us a people, you never talked down to us.

We always had and still today, have your full attention. You are always on our side. You were a loving, tolerant husband, who stood in the background, letting mom be the front man.

You never punished us unjustly, and then when it was time, you let us go into the world and experience life for ourselves. There were times you pushed us. I know now it was because you wanted more for us. I know you must have regrets about your life, dreams unfulfilled, but we never knew it.

Mom loved you with all her heart. She was strong because of you. I always thought, until mom died, that she was the strong one of you two, and I worried what would happen to you when her time came.

But after she died, I saw a strength to you I have never seen before, and I realized it has been you all these years, the quiet one, that was the strong one. You have come through, and continued to live, despite losing your soul mate of 37 years, from a 17 year-old boy, the only constant in your life. You amazed me and continue to.

I am in awe of how you got out of bed and continued living, knowing the hurt was overwhelming, and the relief was causing you guilt. You persevered, and you showed us that is what mom wanted. That was where you could truly honor your time with mom, was to continue on, for us. You are an amazing "Bobbu," dad and father in law, and man.

When you found out about my test results, you were always there, never telling me what to do. You trusted that I knew what I was doing, and, though I sheltered you at times from the truth of my feelings, you were always there reminding me often of how much you loved me and how proud you were of me.

I thank you, Dad, for it all.

I love you.

Tracy

A LETTER TO MY SISTER

Tammy,

No one knows a life lived like a sibling. No one shares love like a sister. You were always a thorn in my side growing up, let's face it. You were always around, always dependant on me for your social life, your target for tattling. You were always a fighter. I always remember you around. Just like now, as we are adults, you are always there.

You are one of the most giving people I know. Never hesitating to be there for someone in need. Never begrudging them your time.

We went through this together, from the blood test we took side by side, to the results we shared holding hands, to the waiting at the hospital for surgeries to be done, to bringing me "feel better" presents!

There was never resentment, jealousy, or anger about the results between us. You kept me laughing, and never questioned my decision, as you were prepared to do the same.

I know you probably wished it was you, not wanting it to be me. I know you would have done it with me if you could have, and I know you tried to take Mom's place, being there for me when she couldn't. You wore two hats through this, and I noticed and love you for that.

You, now, are the glue that plans the family events, ensures we are doing things together, as mom always did, fearing that if you don't, we will go our separate ways and lose that togetherness. At times when we were young, you fought so hard to get away from all that!

You never wanted to do stuff as a family, always rebelled against it, and now you are fighting for it. What a change. How you have grown, into a strong, confident, stubborn woman!

You hold it together stronger than anyone I know. You are the director in the family, the true fighter in the family, fighting for us. Sorry to tell you, but you have become mom!

I am thankful mom gave you to me. You are the greatest gift she ever gave me.

I Love You.

Tracy xo

A LETTER TO THE READER

As you come to finishing this memoir, although you yourself may not be faced with cancer, you may be faced with other challenges or life altering decisions. Whatever they may be, my book carries the same message to all. In saying that, there are a few things I hope that you take with you as you close it and put it on the shelf.

Trust yourself.

Listen to your gut.

Search for knowledge. Always.

Live with a positive attitude. Always.

Allow yourself to feel whatever it may be that you are going through. You need to feel it to move toward resolution, to a better place.

You need to find what gives you that resolution. Some read, some pray, some exercise, and some, like myself, need to write. Doing these things will lead you to resolution, to a place you weren't and can't get to in your moment of emotion, but can truly only get to after you experience all the feelings that come with the challenge you face.

I thank you for taking time out of your life, to read about my journey.

Remember, knowledge is power, so take whatever helps you from whatever page you found it.

I wish you many footprints in your sand as you face moments of "what now" on your life's journey.

In this battle we are all in against breast cancer, we will one day all stand together cheering, celebrating, crying and rejoicing, because collectively we would have all contributed to the cure for breast cancer. That day is coming.

"Never, never, never give up. Never."

Winston Churchill

Printed in the United States
125081LV00003B/151-249/P